INNER INSIGHTS

THE BOOK OF CHARTS

Alternative Medicine & Awareness
Quick Reference Charts

Linda Mackenzie

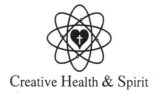

Creative Health & Spirit

Creative Health & Spirit
P.O. Box 385
Manhattan Beach, CA 90267

This book is manufactured in the United States of America.

Library of Congress Catalog Number: 97-91455

Inner Insights - The Book of Chart: Alternative Medicine & Awareness
Quick Reference Charts/ by Linda Mackenzie

Includes Index   Bibliography: p
ISBN # 0- 9656432-1-2   (Trade Paper Edition)
1. Self Help   2. Reference   3. Alternative Medicine   4. Spiritual Life
5. Philosophy   6. New Age   I.Title

Acknowledgments

It is with gratitude and respect that I acknowledge all those whose writings and efforts have aided in the research of this book. To all the authors and philosophers throughout the centuries, I express my thanks - for without their prior research and knowledge this book would not have been possible.

I wish to express my heartfelt appreciation to:

Lisa, my daughter, whose patience I'm sure was tried at times, yet always did she love and support me.

All my family and friends whose never ending encouragement gave me the fortitude to realize my dream and make it a reality.

But most of all to God, who has blessed my life with many gifts and has given me the ability to reach people and help them on their path to enlightenment.

THIS BOOK IS DEDICATED TO
ALL SEEKERS OF SELF-DISCOVERY.

My goal is to support you in your search for increased self awareness and informed insight into life's challenges. By serving as a resource for your own personal quest I hope this book becomes an uplifting force in your life.

I believe that the positive aspects of life and health become a personal reality as each of us raises our own level of consciousness to be the best that we can be in -
Body, Mind & Spirit.

Therefore what better dedication than to you, my readers. I wish you a life filled with Balance, Clarity and Strength.

Table of Contents

INTRODUCTION

Have you ever wondered about what your Zodiac sign means? How about what herb you could use for a specific illness or what animals mean in your dreams? The quick reference charts in this book are designed to give you answers to your questions on over 40 Alternative Medicine and Awareness subjects. The book provides a wealth of information on general and little known facts at a glance.

There were several reasons why I compiled this book of charts. In this Information Age we need facts fast. Therefore, a book of charts, in an easy to read format, seemed to be able to fulfill this need. We also need to increase our knowledge on subjects that can keep us healthy and aid in our self-discovery process. The chart subjects have been selected for this very purpose. The last reason and perhaps the most important one is that we deserve some fun. Whether you take the information seriously or not, it is fun to discover what our favorite color means or what animal represents us in the Chinese Horoscope.

The charts in the book are Quick Reference Charts, those interested in further detail, are encouraged to obtain specific books on the topics that interest them. I have provided a Reading List that I have found useful in my explorations.

The information in the charts was derived from many cultures, over many centuries. The meanings I have chosen are generally accepted "standards". If you run across discrepancies in other books, I encourage you not to judge any "standards" and be open to what is right for you. Use your intuition, your gut feel and expand your mind. You really are the only person who knows what's right for you.

For convenience the charts are presented in alphabetical order. Although some of the chart topics may be familiar to you, others may not. Have fun and explore them all. I have provided some short general explanations per topic to get you started on your road to self discovery.

List of Charts

Acupressure Applications   **Related Healing Points and Common Ailment Applications**
A selection of common ailments and their related acupressure healing points are shown. According to Eastern tradition if you apply pressure on the appropriate point for 7-10 seconds, symptoms can be relieved and energy balance is restored.

Acupressure Points   **Illustration of Major Points Front/Back View**
According to Eastern tradition energy is believed to flow through the body in specific paths. When a blockage occurs in the energy flow path illness or mental disorders result. By applying pressure to an associated "point" symptoms can be relieved.

Angels - Hierarchy   **Divine Hierarchical Order and Ruling Angels**
An angel is a "pure and divine spirit", a "messenger", a "ministering or guiding spirit" and according to the scriptures employed by God. The three Hierarchies and nine choirs are shown. A list of Ruling Angels of the days, months, planets, elements, winds, Sephirah and Zodiac are provided.

Angels - Specialties   **Rank, Attributes and Specialties of the Angels**
Angels are prevalent in many religions. Some say that even plant and animals have an angel. The first chart alphabetically lists the angel name, rank and attributes. The second chart lists the angel name and their specialty.

Aromatherapy   **Names, Uses, Results and Application Methods**
By using or combining certain plant oils, the "aroma" can become a "therapy to relieve mental and physical discomforts. Some of the basic Aromatherapy oils, what they are used for and how to use them are given.

Astrology   **Information on all 12 Zodiac Signs**
The basis of Astrology is the study of the Zodiac (an imaginary belt in the heavens) and the related positions of the planets, moon and sun at the time of your birth. Astrology can tell the story of your life path. Divided into twelve Zodiac signs, general and little known facts are provided for each sign.

Auras   **Attributes and Qualities of the Energies**
Auras are atmospheres of energy arise and surround the body. These Auras have particular colors, qualities, and attributes.

Bach Flowers   **Problem Traits, Flower Application and Result**
A Holistic remedy for emotional problems, Bach Flowers are comprised of specific flower tinctures which are distilled into a tonic or drops. These drops and tinctures are taken internally to benefit emotional distress.

Cabala - Tree of Life   Name, Source, Qualities and attributes of the Sephirah

In a faction of the Jewish religion, the Cabala (also known as Kabala or Kabbala) is considered the Tree of Life. The Cabala diagram sketches out a blueprint of how the energy of life may be experienced. Energy is said to flow from top to bottom of the Tree. The balance and relationship of the Sephirah is the basis of the Tree of Life.

Card Fortune Telling   Ancient Divination Method

Cards are an ancient method of tapping into the subconscious mind to see the potential and possibilities of your situation. This provides insight into making the right decisions. Using a deck of ordinary playing cards and this chart you can find answers to questions.

The Major Chakras   Name, Location, Qualities and Attributes of the Chakras

The major Chakras "the esoteric energy centers of the body" are comprised of seven energy centers found in specific locations in the body. Energy flows through these centers and is said to influence emotions, health, thought, intuition, psychic abilities and creativity.

Cheyenne Medicine Wheel   Directions, Attributes and Meanings

In Native American Tradition the Cheyenne Medicine Wheel depicts the Wheel of Life. Everyone walks the wheel to raise consciousness, gain power and facilitate growth experiences. The energy centers of the Wheel are the Four Directions.

Chinese Elements   Elements, Qualities and Attributes

The Chinese Elements are the forces of Nature that can be expressed as a primary influence of life forces. There are five elements that characterize the life cycle - Birth, Initiation, Love, Rest and Death.

Chinese Herbs   Names, Parts Utilized and Uses

Chinese Herbs have been a long accepted cure for illness and disease in the East. These herbs are gaining popularity for curing illness and dysfunction in the West. The chart lists the major Chinese Herbs and their uses.

Chinese Horoscope   Signs and Meanings

The Chinese Horoscope has been around for over 2,000 years. Each Chinese New Year is associated with an animal. Legend states that Buddha called all the animals to his side. As each of the twelve animals appeared before Buddha, each animal was assigned a Chinese year in the order of appearance. Your birth year in the Chinese Horoscope determines your Chinese Horoscope sign.

Color   Aspects, Qualities and Attributes of Color

Each color has it's own energy qualities that effect our mind, body and spirit. By recognizing the different colors you are drawn to you can recognize where you are in your body-mind-spirit. If a color is not listed, combine the two or three colors that up your desired color and read those meanings.

Favorite Colors
Favorite Colors and their Personality Meanings

Color can psychologically effect us for many different reasons. For example, through past learned reactions, cultural attitudes, climate (each season has it's own dawn to dusk characteristics) or income level (all economic groups use color to reflect status within a group) you may have certain likes and dislikes about certain colors. The colors you like or your favorite colors can tell you something about your personality. If you have more than one favorite color your personality traits are the combination of the colors you like.

Healing Colors
Healing Color, Color Activation & Uses

Spectral colors have been shown to aid the body in healing. By applying color to specific areas of the body through a colored light therapy called Radionics it has been stated that it may help in healing.

Healing Colors & Music
Healing Color Qualities and Musical Notes

Pythagoreanism is a philosophy which believes in the migration of the soul and that numbers are the primary elements of the Universe. A part of the Pythagorean theory is that each color is associated with a musical note. Because musical notes produce vibrations to the ears and colors produce vibrations to the eyes we manifest a physical reaction to color and sound. If we apply the appropriate color/sound vibrations they can change our emotional state and aid in healing the body.

Crystals & Gemstones
Favorite Colors and their Personality Meanings

Each particular stone vibrates it's own energy and has spiritual and healing properties. If we carry or wear a stone we perpetrate our own energies and pave the way to getting our desired results. Whether those results are enhanced enlightenment, healing or coping with life on earth stones can help us. The chart lists crystals, gemstones, metals & ores.

Dice Fortune Telling
Answers to Questions and Future Revelations

The method of using Dice for divination was used for centuries in India and China. Allowing us to access our subconscious mind Dice can help you discern answers about life and your future.

Domino Fortune Telling
Answers to Questions and Future Revelations

Dominoes are an Ancient Tradition Method from China to give answers about life questions and provide a look into what the future might hold.

Gods - Names & Origins
Names, Origins and Descriptions

This chart alphabetically lists the names of Gods, their country of origin and a brief description about them.

Goddess Circle of Power
Directions and their Meanings, Attributes & Power

The energy centers in the Circle of Power are the Four Directions. Each direction relates to a mind-body-universe connection, has a specific time, color, element, animal & power.

Goddesses - Names & Origins   Names, Origins and Descriptions

This chart alphabetically lists the names of Goddesses, their country of origin and a brief description about them.

Goddess Symbols   Symbols and their Meanings

Since primitive man there have been many symbols that have related to Goddesses. Whether it is an animal, bird, circle, etc. each symbol has a specific meaning.

I Ching - Coin Toss   Divination Method and Meanings

The I Ching comes from China and takes a look at human behavior in relationship to the elements. Action or change is considered to affect the individual action and the universe. The coin toss method is very old and provides insight with key words. I encourage people who are interested to read more about this subject.

I Ching Trigrams   Meanings and Cyclic trigram Arrangement

The I Ching or Book of Changes has been used for over 3,000 years. This philosophical system is based on quantum physics and mathematics. A Hexagram is a six line structure comprised of solid/broken lines. There are 64 Hexagrams used. Two Trigrams, each a three line structure, make up a Hexagram. There are eight Trigrams. These Trigrams have meanings and a cyclic Cycle.

NA Animal Dream Spirits   Meanings of Animals in Your Dreams

According to Native American Indian Tradition, if an animal appears in your dreams it has a meaning or is trying to tell you something.

NA Animal Spirit Communication   Animals and their Meanings

In the Native American Indian Tradition if an animal crosses your path they have a meaning or a message for you.

Numerology   Numbers, Symbols, Cycles, Aspects & Meanings

Numerology uses the scientific aspect of numerical measurement to give insight into ourselves and people around us.

Palm Reading   General Meanings

Palmistry is a method of telling a person about his traits and future. This is based upon the interpretation of hand type, main lines, mounts, markings and line traits.

Phrenology   Head Areas and Meanings

There is method of determining personality traits by examining the bumps on your head. Each area of the head rules a particular aspect of a person. If a bump is found in a specific area, the area's qualities/meanings can give you insight into the personality.

Planets   Symbols, Attributes, Qualities and Meanings

The planets have long been a source of interest and mystery. This chart provides a collection of scientific and esoteric facts about each planet.

Reflexology   Bottom, Side and Top Points

Reflexologists believe that all parts of the body has a corresponding pressure point on the feet. By applying pressure or rubbing the feet in a specific area you can relieve symptoms from ailments and illness.

Runes   Rune Signs, Aspects and Meanings

Runes are the spiritual alphabet of the Ancient Northern European people. Each rune has a symbol and is used for decision making, enlightenment and guidance.

The Seven Rays   Color and Meanings

Alice Bailey provided a theory that Infinity is a white brilliance that refracts energy into seven rays of light. Two rays are said to dominate each life. The first ray dominates the soul and the second the personality.

Sioux Four Directions   Directions and their Meanings

The energy centers of Life are located in the Four directions. These directions have meanings that raise awareness, provide power and facilitate growth experiences.

Palm Reading   General Meanings

Palmistry is a method of telling a person about his traits and future. This is based upon the interpretation of hand type, main lines, mounts, markings and line traits.

The Tarot   Meanings and Associations

The Tarot is an Ancient Tradition method performed with a Pictorial Deck of Cards to gain insight into life questions and future revelations. The chart gives the qualities, life cycle, music, chakra, astrology, planet, archetype and meanings of all twenty-two cards.

Tea Leaf Reading   Symbols and their Meanings

Reading tea leaves is a method to get answers to questions and the future. Certain preparations are used to enable the reading of the tea leaf symbols. Symbols are interpreted by the reader and their meanings and interpretations can vary.

Vitamins & Minerals   Body Activity and Uses

Vitamins, minerals and supplements are important to maintain a healthy body. Lists the the major vitamins, minerals and supplements, their effect on body activity and their uses.

Western Elements   Elements, Qualities and Attributes

Elements are the forces of Nature that can be expressed as a primary influence of life force. The four Western Elements have qualities, aspects and associations.

THE CHARTS

ACUPRESSURE APPLICATIONS

SYMPTOM	BLADDER	CONCEPTION VESSEL	GALL BLADDER	GOVERNING VESSEL	HEART	KIDNEY	LARGE INTESTINE	LIVER	LUNG	PERICARDIUM	SMALL INTESTINES	STOMACH	SPLEEN	TRIPLE WARMER
ANXIETY					5, 7				1, 2			42	3	
ASTHMA	38	17			3, 8				1, 2					
BACK PAIN	38, 45, 48			2, 4										
BLADDER	60, 64, 66, 67													
CLAUSTROPHOBIA					5, 7, 8, 9				1, 2	5, 8		42	3	
CONGESTION	48	17							1, 2			1		
CONJUNCTIVITIS	1, 2		1					3					7	
CONSTIPATION							4					40, 45*		
DEPRESSION					5, 7, 8, 9	1*	1		1, 2	8				
EAR DISCOMFORT	64					1*								
FATIGUE						1*, 3, 11, 22						36		
FEVER	66				7	8				7	4		3	4
GAS									1, 9			45	1*, 3	
GOUT	2				7				1, 2			42		
HEADACHE - FRONT			1, 14	4							-	6		23
HEADACHE - SIDES			4, 20								19	6, 7		23
HEADACHE - BACK			19, 20	17							-	-		16, 19
HEARTBURN												42	4	
HERPES	66												7	
HOT FLASHES						3						42		3
IMPOTENCE		2		14	7, 9	1, 3, 7, 11				8				1
INSOMNIA					7, 9	3, 8			1					
MENSTRUAL CRAMPS		2										36, 42	3, 46, 10, 12	
NAUSEA												42	3	
SORE THROAT		24												
PROSTRATE	64	6			1, 3									
SHOCK		17			7, 9	1*			1, 2	5				
STRESS		17			7, 9				1, 2		10*	42		
TOOTHACHE				28										
VOMITING												42	3	

* Not To Be Used When Pregnant.

ACUPRESSURE APPLICATIONS

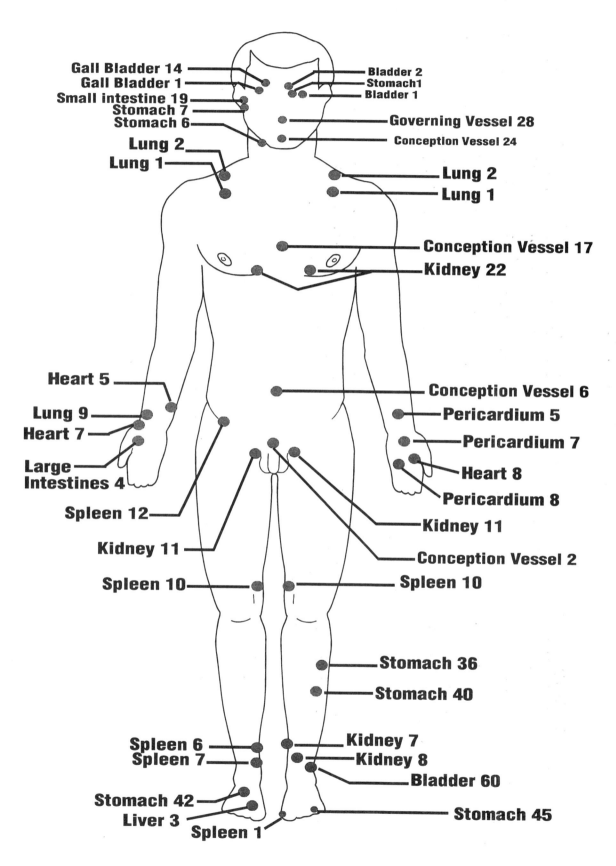

Gall Bladder 14
Gall Bladder 1
Small intestine 19
Stomach 7
Stomach 6
Lung 2
Lung 1

Bladder 2
Stomach 1
Bladder 1
Governing Vessel 28
Conception Vessel 24
Lung 2
Lung 1

Conception Vessel 17
Kidney 22

Heart 5
Lung 9
Heart 7
Large Intestines 4
Spleen 12
Kidney 11
Spleen 10

Conception Vessel 6
Pericardium 5
Pericardium 7
Heart 8
Pericardium 8
Kidney 11
Conception Vessel 2
Spleen 10

Stomach 36
Stomach 40

Spleen 6
Spleen 7
Stomach 42
Liver 3
Spleen 1

Kidney 7
Kidney 8
Bladder 60
Stomach 45

ACUPRESSURE POINTS

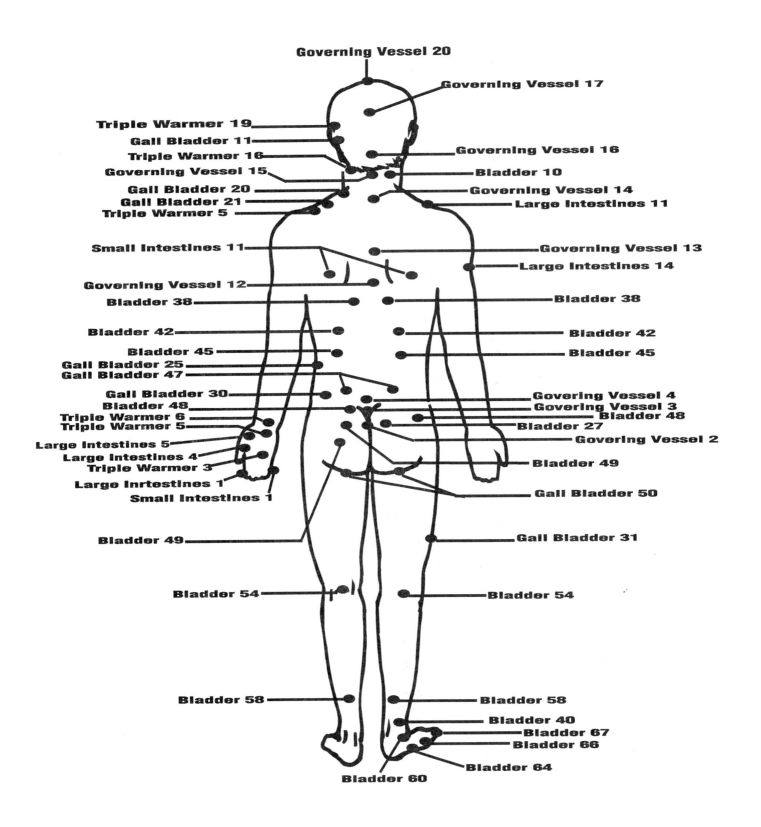

Governing Vessel 20

Governing Vessel 17

Triple Warmer 19

Gall Bladder 11

Triple Warmer 16

Governing Vessel 15

Gall Bladder 20

Gall Bladder 21

Triple Warmer 5

Small Intestines 11

Governing Vessel 12

Bladder 38

Bladder 42

Bladder 45

Gall Bladder 25

Gall Bladder 47

Gall Bladder 30

Bladder 48

Triple Warmer 6

Triple Warmer 5

Large Intestines 5

Large Intestines 4

Triple Warmer 3

Large Inrtestines 1

Small Intestines 1

Bladder 49

Bladder 54

Bladder 58

Governing Vessel 16

Bladder 10

Governing Vessel 14

Large Intestines 11

Governing Vessel 13

Large Intestines 14

Bladder 38

Bladder 42

Bladder 45

Goverring Vessel 4

Goverring Vessel 3

Bladder 48

Bladder 27

Goverring Vessel 2

Bladder 49

Gall Bladder 50

Gall Bladder 31

Bladder 54

Bladder 58

Bladder 40

Bladder 67

Bladder 66

Bladder 64

Bladder 60

ACUPRESSURE POINTS

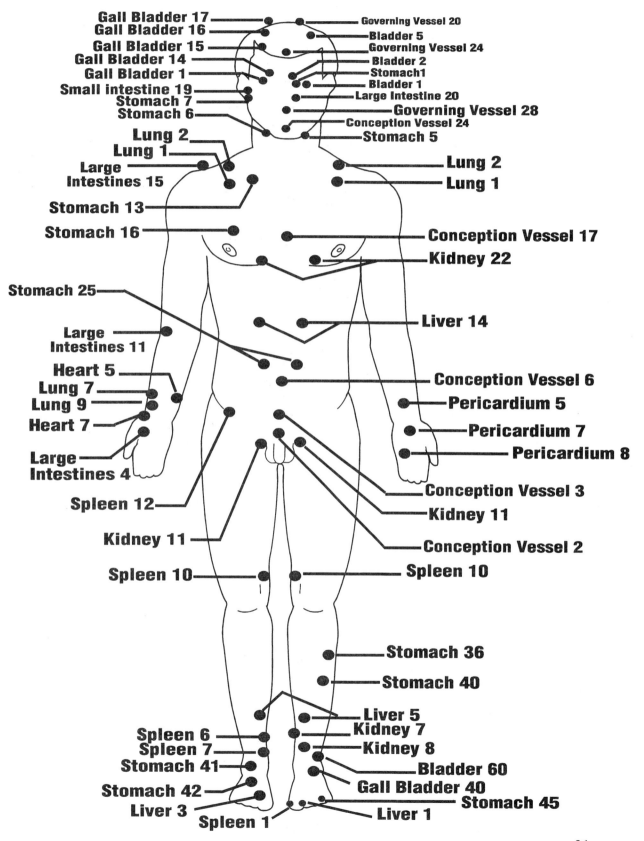

Gall Bladder 17
Gall Bladder 16
Gall Bladder 15
Gall Bladder 14
Gall Bladder 1
Small intestine 19
Stomach 7
Stomach 6
Lung 2
Lung 1
Large Intestines 15
Stomach 13
Stomach 16
Stomach 25
Large Intestines 11
Heart 5
Lung 7
Lung 9
Heart 7
Large Intestines 4
Spleen 12
Kidney 11
Spleen 10
Governing Vessel 20
Bladder 5
Governing Vessel 24
Bladder 2
Stomach1
Bladder 1
Large Intestine 20
Governing Vessel 28
Conception Vessel 24
Stomach 5
Lung 2
Lung 1
Conception Vessel 17
Kidney 22
Liver 14
Conception Vessel 6
Pericardium 5
Pericardium 7
Pericardium 8
Conception Vessel 3
Kidney 11
Conception Vessel 2
Spleen 10
Stomach 36
Stomach 40
Liver 5
Kidney 7
Kidney 8
Bladder 60
Gall Bladder 40
Stomach 45
Spleen 6
Spleen 7
Stomach 41
Stomach 42
Liver 3
Spleen 1
Liver 1

31

ANGELS HIERARCHY

HIERARCHY 1

SERAPHIM - CHOIR 1
SPIRITS OF LOVE & POSITIVE UNIVERSE

MICHAEL KEMEUL JEHOEL
SERAPHIEL URIEL METATRON
NATHANAEL

RESIDENCE: CLOSEST TO GOD

CHERUBIM - CHOIR 2
SPIRITS OF HARMONY - WISDOM OF GOD

GABRIEL RAPHAEL ZOPHIEL
CHERUBIEL OPHANIEL

RESIDENCE: FIXED STARS

THRONES - CHOIR 3
SPIRITS OF WILL & JUSTICE

ORIFIE JAPHAKIEL RAZIEL
BARADIEL ZAPHKIEL

RESIDENCE: SATURN

HIERARCHY 2

DOMINIONS - CHOIR 1
SPIRITS OF WISDOM & INTUITION

ZADKIEL HASMAEL
MURIEL ZACHAREL

RESIDENCE: JUPITER

VIRTUES - CHOIR 2
SPIRITS OF CHOICE & MOVEMENT

UZZIEL HANIEL MICHAEL
BABIEL PEUEL GABRIEL
TARSHIEL

RESIDENCE: MARS

POWERS - CHOIR 3
SPIRITS OF FORM & SPACE

RAPHAEL CAMAEL VERCHIEL

RESIDENCE: SUN

HIERARCHY 3

PRINCIPALITIES - CHOIR 1
SPIRITS OF PERSONALITY & TIME

URIEL ANAEL MICHAEL
RAGUEL RAPHAEL GABRIEL
REMIEL

RESIDENCE: VENUS

ARCHANGELS - CHOIR 2
SPIRITS OF FIRE, RULING ANGELS

MICHAEL RAPHAEL REMIEL
URIEL GABRIEL RAGUEL
SARIEL

RESIDENCE: MERCURY

ANGELS - CHOIR 3
SPIRITS OF NATURE, MESSENGERS

MULTITUDES THAT ARE INTERMEDIARIES
BETWEEN GOD & HUMANS

RESIDENCE: MOON

GUARDIAN ANGELS
GUARDIAN SPIRITS OF HUMAN BEINGS

EVERYONE HAS THEIR OWN PERSONAL
ANGEL ASSIGNED AT BIRTH FOR THEIR
PROTECTION.

RESIDENCE: NEAR HUMAN BODY IN LIFE

ZODIAC ANGELS

ARIES - MACHIDIEL
TAURUS - ASMODEL
GEMINI - AMBRIEL
CANCER - MURIEL

LEO - VERCHIEL
VIRGO - HAMALIEL
LIBRA - URIEL
SCORPIO - BARBIEL

SAGITTARRIUS- ADNACHIEL
CAPRICORN -HANAEL
AQUARIUS - GABRIEL
PISCES - BARCHIEL

32

ANGELS HIERARCHY

ARCHANGELS & ANGELS OF THE SEVEN DAYS

	SUNDAY	MONDAY	TUESDAY	WEDNESDAY	THURSDAY	FRIDAY	SATURDAY
ARCHANGELS	RAPHAEL	GABRIEL	KHAMAEL	MICHAEL	TZAPHIEL	HANIEL	TZAPHIEL
ANGELS	MICHAEL	GABRIEL	ZAMUEL	RAPHAEL	SACHIEL	ANAEL	CASSIEL

PLANET ANGELS

SUN-RAPHAEL   MOON-GABRIEL
VENUS-ARIEL   SATURN-KAFZIEL
MERCURY- MICHAEL   MARS-SAMMAEL
JUPITER-ZADKIEL

ELEMENT & WIND ANGELS

FIRE- NATHANIEL   NORTH WIND-GABRIEL
AIR-CHERUB   SOUTH WIND-URIEL
WATER-THARSIS   EAST WIND-MICHAEL
EARTH-ARIEL   WEST WIND-RAPHAEL

ANGELS OF THE MONTHS

JANUARY	GABRIEL
FEBRUARY	BARCHIEL
MARCH	MACHIDIEL
APRIL	ASMODEL
MAY	AMBRIEL
JUNE	MURIEL
JULY	VERCHIEL
AUGUST	HAMALIEL
SEPTEMBER	URIEL
OCTOBER	BARBIEL
NOVEMBER	ADNACHIEL
DECEMBER	HANAEL

ANGELS OF THE SEPHIRAH (KABBALA)

KETHER (CROWN)	METATRON
CHOKMAH (WISDOM)	RAZIEL
BINAH (UNDERSTANDING)	TZAPHQIEL
CHESED (MERCY)	TZADQIEL
GEBURAH (STRENGTH)	KHAMAEL
TIPERETH (BEAUTY)	MICHAEL
NETZACH (VICTORY)	HANIEL
HOD (SPLENDOR)	RAPHAEL
JESOD (FOUNDATION)	GABRIEL
MALKUTH (KINGDOM)	METATRON

ANGEL ATTRIBUTES

NAME	RANK/ATTRIBUTES	NAME	RANK/ATTRIBUTES
ANAEL	Principality / Fertility, Human Sexuality	PELIEL	Virtue / Courage, Grace, Movement, Choice
AZRAEL	Destruction / Sword of God, Help of God Angel of Death	RAGUEL	Principality, Archangel / Ruling Angel, Personality, Time, Religion Protector
BABIEL	Virtue / Courage, Grace	RAPHAEL	Cherub, Power, Principality, Archangel / Ruling Angel, Harmony, Intellect, Healer, Guards the Earth,
BARADIEL	Throne / Wisdom of God	RAZIEL	Throne / Will, Judgement
CAMAEL	Power / Intellect, Defeats Devils, Mathematics, Geometry	REMIEL	Principality, Archangel / Ruling Angel God's Messanger
CASSIEL	Joy	RHAIMIEL	(St. Francis of Assisi) Mercy, Kindness
CHERUBIEL	Cherub / Wisdom of God, Harmony	SACHIEL	Protection
GABRIEL	Cherub, Virtue, Principality, Archangel / Ruling Angel, Man of God, Comfort, Understanding, Vengeance	SANASIEL	Gate of Life, Prays for Souls
HANIEL	Virtue / Courage, Grace Favor of God	SARIEL	Sword of God, Defeats Evil
HASMAL	Dominion / Wisdom, Intuition	SERAPHIEL	Seraph / Love & Positive Spirit, Nearest to God
JAPHKIEL	Throne / Will, Justice	SIMIKIEL	Sword of God
JEHOEL	Seraph / Angel of Fire, Ruling Angel Singer of the Eternal	TARSHISH	Virtue / Movement, Choice, Grace, Courage
KEMEUL	Seraph / Helper of God, Mediator	URIEL	Seraph, Principality, Archangel / Ruling Angel Power of God, Love, Time, Personality
METATRON	Archangel / Chancellor of Heaven Sustenance of Mankind	UZZIEL	Virtue / Power of God, Movement, Choice, Courage, Grace
MICHAEL	Seraph, Virtue, Principality, Archangel / Ruling Angel, Like Unto God, Truth, Strength, Mercy, Rescues Souls	VERCHIEL	Power / Form, Space, Intellect, Defeats Devils, Geometry
MURIEL	Dominion / Wisdom, Intuition	ZACHARIEL	Dominion / Guardian of Order, Wisdom
NATHANAEL	Seraph / Love & Positive Spirit, Gift of God, Hidden Things	ZADKIEL	Dominion / Mercy, Wisdom, Intuition
OPHANIEL	Cherub / Harmony, Wisdom of God	ZAPHKIEL	Throne / Will, Justice
ORIFIEL	Throne / Will, Justice	ZEHANPUYU	Messenger of Mercy
PENIEL	Face of God, Cures Human Stupidity	ZOPHEL	Cherub / Harmony, Wisdom

ANGEL SPECIALTIES

ANGEL OF:/ NAME	ANGEL OF:/ NAME	ANGEL OF:/ NAME
ANNUNCIATION/GABRIEL	FOOD/MANNA	MUSIC/ISRAFIL
APOCALYPSE/ORIFIEL	FORESTS/ZUPHLAS	PATIENCE/ACHAIAH
ASPIRATION/GABRIEL	FORGETFULLNESS/POTEH	POETRY/URIEL
BALANCE/MICHAEL	FREE WILL/TABRIS	PROGRESS/RAPHAEL
BEASTS (TAME)/HARIEL	FUTURE/ISIAIEL	PURITY/TAHARIEL
BEASTS (WILD)/THURIEL	GRACE/ANANCHEL	REVELATION/GABRIEL
BENEVOLENCE/ZADKIEL	HEALING/RAPHAEL	RIGHTEOUSNESS/MICHAEL
BIRDS/ARAEL	HOLY SPIRIT/GABRIEL	SCIENCE/RAPHAEL
CHANCE/URIEL	HOPE/PHANUEL	SEA/TAMIEL
COMPASSION/RAPHAEL	INVENTIONS/LIWET	SKY/SAHAQIEL
CONCEPTION/LAILA	JOY/RAPHAEL	SOLITUTDE/CASSIEL
DAYLIGHT/SAMSHIEL	JUDGEMENT/GABRIEL	SOULS OF MEN/REMIEL
SEA/RAMPEL	JUSTICE/TSADKIEL	STRENGTH/ZERUCH
DESTINY/ORIEL	KNOWLEDGE/RAPHAEL	THUNDER/URIEL
DIVINATION/EISTIBUS	LOVE/THELIEL	TREES/MAKTIEL
DREAMS/GABRIEL	MANKIND/METATRON	TRUTH/MICHAEL
EARTHQUAKES/RASHIEL	MEMORY/ZADKIEL	TRUTH/GABRIEL
FATE/MANU	MERCY/RAHMIEL	VICTORY/BAHRAM
FIRE/NATHANIEL	MORALS/MEHABIAH	WAR/MICHAEL,GABRRIEL
FISH/GAGIEL	MOUNTAINS/RAMPEL	WATER/THARSIS

AROMATHERAPY

NAME	USED FOR	USE AS:
BASIL	ANXIETY, NERVES, MENTAL FATIGUE	I
BERGAMOT	ANXIETY, DEPRESSION, ECZEMA, DERMATITIS	M, B, V
CEDAR	PAST EMOTIONAL PAIN	I
CHAMOMILE	ANGER, DIGESTION, OVERWORK, IRRITATION	M, B, I
EUCALYPTUS	COLDS, BRONCHITIS, ARTHRITIS, MUSCLE PAIN INFECTIONS, IMMUNE DEFICIENCY	M, I, V
EVENING PRIMROSE OIL	NERVOUS DISORDERS, PMS, CIRCULATION, REPRODUCTIVE BALANCE	M, I, ME
FRANKINCENSE	NIGHTMARES, FEAR, RHEMATOID ARTHRITIS	M, B, V
GERANIUM	MOOD SWINGS, ULCERS, MENOPAUSE, DIARRHEA	M, B, P, ME
GINGER	STRAINED MUSCLES	M, B, I
GRAPEFRUIT	DEPRESSION, RESENTMENT, GALL STONES, KIDNEY STONES, ARTERY DEPOSITS	M, B, P, ME, V
JASMINE	DEPRESSION, LACK OF CONFIDENCE, FRIGIDITY, IMPOTENCE, EMOTIONAL COLDNESS, INTROVERT	M, B, P, V, I
JUNIPER	CYSTITIS, URINARY INFECTIONS, GOUT, CRAMPS, ARTHRITIS, PAST EMOTIONAL PAIN	M, ME
LAVENDER	ANXIETY, INSOMNIA, BURNS, INSECT BITES, SENSUAL STIMULANT, ECZEMA, ANTISEPTIC	M, B, P, I, V
LEMON GRASS	SPIRITUAL PROTECTION	M, B, I
MARJORAM	ANXIETY, STRESS, HYPERTENSION, INSOMNIA, HEADACHES, PANIC ATTACKS,	M, B, I
M=MASSAGE B=BATH V=VAPORIZER I=INHALATION P=PERFUME ME=MEDICINE		

AROMATHERAPY

NAME	USED FOR	USE AS:
NEROLI	STRESS DUE TO DEPRESSION, SADNESS	I
ORANGE BLOSSOM	ANXIETY, STRESS, PALPITATIONS, INSOMNIA, IMMUNE DEFICIENCY	M, B, P, V, I
PATCHOULI	SENSUAL STIMULANT	B, I
PEPPERMINT	DIGESTION, MEMORY, CONGESTION, NAUSEA, PURIFICATION, MUSCLE/JOINT PAIN, MENTAL FATIGUE	M, B, I, ME, V
PINE	CONGESTION, RESPIRATORY	B, I
ROSE	ANXIETY, EMOTIONAL TRAUMA, IMPATIENCE, CONFUSION, SENSUAL STIMULANT, HEART SORROW	M, B, P
ROSEMARY	MENTAL FATIGUE, MEMORY, ARTHRITIS, IMMUNE DEFICIENCY, CONGESTION, ACHES	M, B, V, I
ROSE OTTO	DEPRESSION, GRIEF, HANG OVERS	M, B, P
SAGE	DEPRESSION, CRAMPS, THROAT INFECTIONS, LARYNGITIS, SPIRITUAL PURIFICATION	M, B, P, V, I
SANDALWOOD	STRESS, FEAR, INSECURITY, LARYNGITIS, URINARY INFECTIONS, THROAT INFECTIONS	M, B, I, ME, V
SPIKENARD	SPIRITUAL PROTECTION	B, I
TEA TREE	BURNS, INSECT BITES, ATHLETE'S FOOT, RINGWORM, THRUSH, CYSTITIS, NAIL INFECTIONS	M, ME
THYME	MUSCLE STRAINS	M, B, I
YLANG YLANG	DEPRESSION, ANGER, IMPOTENCE, FRIGIDY, HYPERTENSION, PALPITATIONS	M, B, P, V, I

M=MASSAGE B=BATH V=VAPORIZER I=INHALATION P=PERFUME ME=MEDICINE

ASTROLOGY

SIGN	SYMBOL	ELEMENT	PLANET	HOUSE	POLARITY/ QUALITY	COLOR	STONES
ARIES ♈ 3/21-4/20 "I AM"	RAM	FIRE	MARS	1ST	POSITIVE\ CARDINAL	BRIGHT RED	DIAMOND GARNET RUBY
TAURUS ♉ 4/21-5/21 "I HAVE"	BULL CRESCENT MOON	EARTH	VENUS	2ND	NEGATIVE\ FIXED	DEEP BLUE	EMERALD SAPPHIRE ROSE QUARTZ
GEMINI ♊ 5/22-6/21 "I THINK"	TWINS	AIR	MERCURY	3RD	POSITIVE\ MUTABLE	BLUE	TURQUOISE AQUAMARINE CLEAR QUARTZ
CANCER ♋ 6/22-7/23 "I CARE"	CRAB	WATER	MOON	4TH	NEGATIVE\ CARDINAL	GREEN	PEARL, MOONSTONE ALEXANDRITE
LEO ♌ 7/24-8/23 "I PROTECT" "I WILL"	LION	FIRE	SUN	5TH	POSITIVE\ FIXED	ORANGE, YELLOW	TIGER'S EYE TOPAZ CITRINE
VIRGO ♍ 8/24-9/23 "I ANALYZE" "I SERVE"	VIRGIN HARVEST GODDESS SPHINX	EARTH	MERCURY	6TH	NEGATIVE\ MUTABLE	BLUE	AGATE PINK JASPER AMAZONITE
LIBRA ♎ 9/24-10/23 "I HARMONIZE"	SCALES	AIR	VENUS	7TH	POSITIVE\ CARDINAL	PINK, PALE BLUE	OPAL PINK TOURMALINE KUNZITE
SCORPIO ♏ 10/24-11/22 "I DESIRE"	SCORPION CURLED SERPENT PHOENIX	WATER	MARS PLUTO	8TH	NEGATIVE\ FIXED	DEEP RED BLACK	TOPAZ GARNET BLOODSTONE
SAGITTARIUS ♐ 11/23-12/21 "I SEEK" "I SEE"	ARCHER CENTAUR	FIRE	JUPITER	9TH	POSITIVE\ MUTABLE	INDIGO, VIOLET	TURQUOISE LAPIS LAZULI
CAPRICORN ♑ 12/22-1/20 "I USE"	GOAT	EARTH	SATURN	10TH	NEGATIVE\ CARDINAL	BLACK, GREEN	ONYX MALACHITE SMOKY QUARTZ
AQUARIUS ♒ 1/21-2/19 "I KNOW" " I DIFFER"	WATER BEARER	AIR	URANUS SATURN	11TH	POSITIVE\ FIXED	ELECTRIC BLUE	SAPPHIRE AQUAMARINE
PISCES ♓ 2/20-3/20 "I BELIEVE"	FISH	WATER	NEPTUNE JUPITER	12TH	NEGATIVE\ MUTABLE	DEEP PURPLE	AMETHYST

ASTROLOGY

SIGN	BODY PART	MUSICAL NOTE	NUMBER	TAROT	ARCHETYPES	COMPATIBILITY	BIOCHEMICAL SALT
ARIES ♈ 3/21-4/20 "I AM"	HEAD	C	9	THE CHARIOT	HERCULES ATHENA	ARIES, LEO, LIBRA, SAGITARRIUS	POTASSIUM SULPHATE (KALI PHOS.)
TAURUS ♉ 4/21-5/21 "I HAVE"	THROAT NECK	C SHARP D FLAT	6	THE TOWER	KING MINOS APHRODITE	TAURUS, CANCER, LEO, SCORPIO, PISCES, CAPRICORN	SODIUM SULPHATE (NAT. SULPH.)
GEMINI ♊ 5/22-6/21 "I THINK"	SHOULDERS ARMS LUNGS	D	5	THE MAGICIAN	HERMES DIOSCURI	ARIES, LIBRA, SAGITARRIUS	POTASSIUM CHLORIDE (KALI MUR)
CANCER ♋ 6/22-7/23 "I CARE"	STOMACH	D SHARP E FLAT	2, 7	THE EMPRESS	MEDUSA ORPHEUS	TAURUS, CANCER, VIRGO, SCORPIO, PISCES, CAPRICORN	CALCIUM FLUORIDE (CALC. FLUOR.)
LEO ♌ 7/24-8/23 "I PROTECT" "I WILL"	HEART BACK SOLAR PLEXUS	E	1, 4	THE SUN	APOLLO PENELOPE	ARIES, LIBRA, AQUARIUS, TAURUS	MAGNESIUM PHOSPHATE (MAG. PHOS.)
VIRGO ♍ 8/24-9/23 "I ANALYZE" "I SERVE"	INTESTINES	F	5	JUDGEMENT	ISIS MERLIN	TAURUS, CANCER, VIRGO, PISCES, CAPRICORN	POTASSIUM PHOSPHATE (KALI SULPH.)
LIBRA ♎ 9/24-10/23 "I HARMONIZE"	KIDNEYS	F SHARP G FLAT	6	THE LOVERS	APHRODITE ODYSSEUS	ARIES, LEO, LIBRA, SAGITARRIUS, CAPRICORN	SODIUM PHOSPHATE (NAT. PHOS.)
SCORPIO ♏ 10/24-11/22 "I DESIRE"	SEXUAL ORGANS	G	9	HIGH PRIESTESS, DEATH	PERSEPHONE GILGAMESH	TAURUS, CANCER, SCORPIO, PISCES, CAPRICORN	CALCIUM SULPHATE (CALC. SULPH.)
SAGITTARIUS ♐ 11/23-12/21 "I SEEK" "I SEE"	THIGHS	G SHARP A FLAT	3	THE HEIROPHANT	HERCULES ZEUS	ARIES, GEMINI, LEO, AQUARIUS, SAGITARRIUS	SILICIC OXIDE (SILICA)
CAPRICORN ♑ 12/22-1/20 "I USE"	KNEES BONES	A	8	THE TAROT	KING MIDAS PAN	TAURUS, CANCER, SCORPIO, VIRGO, LEO, PISCES	CALCIUM PHOSPHATE (CALC. PHOS.)
AQUARIUS ♒ 1/21-2/19 "I KNOW" " I DIFFER"	NERVOUS & CIRCULATORY SYSTEM	A SHARP B FLAT	4, 1	THE STAR	ATALANTA PETER PAN	ARIES, GEMINI, LEO, AQUARIUS, SAGITARRIUS, LIBRA	SODIUM CHLORIDE (NAT. MUR)
PISCES ♓ 2/20-3/20 "I BELIEVE"	FEET	B	3	TEMPERANCE	DIONYSIS TERESA OF AVILA	TAURUS, CANCER, SCORPIO, VIRGO, LEO, CAPRICORN	IRON PHOSPHATE (FERRUM PHOS.)

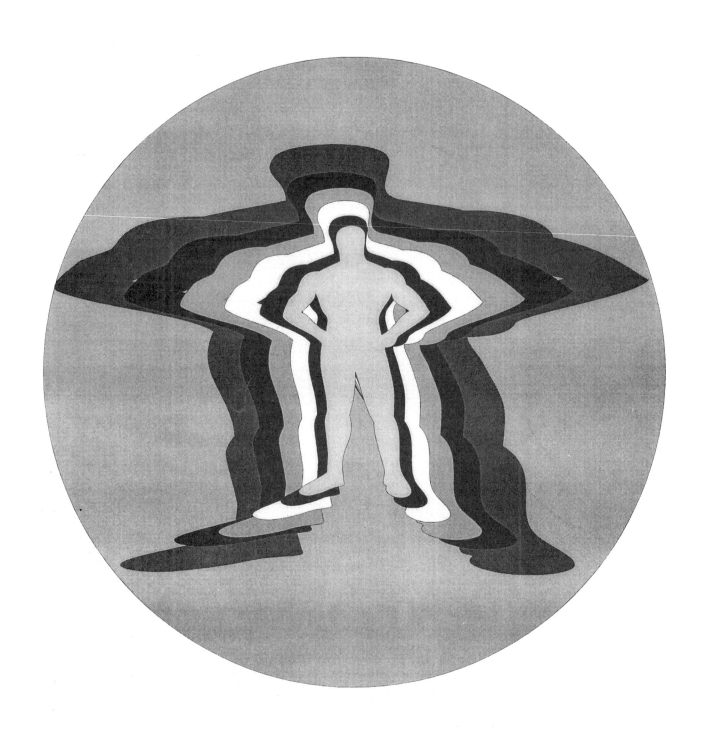

AURAS

BODY	BASE	ENERGY QUALITIES	HUE QUALITIES	SOUND	FEELING	PHRASE
1ST PHYSICAL	EXPERIENCE SENSATION	PHYSICAL MATTER	PHYSICAL BODY	NORMAL SOUND	CONSCIOUSNESS	I EXIST
2ND ETHERIC	KARMA LOVE ASTROLOGICAL	PHYSICAL SENSATION	PALE SHINING BLUE	KEEN HEARING	DEEP PHYSICAL EXPERIENCE	I RESPOND
3RD MENTAL	RATIONAL THOUGHT UNIVERSAL MIND MENTAL PROCESS	PARTITIONED PLANES	YELLOW LIGHT	RYTHMIC BEAT	LOGICAL UNATTACHED EXPERIENCE	I THINK
4TH ASTRAL	DESIRE EMOTION OUT OF BODY TRAVEL	TIMELESSNESS SENSITIVITY CHANGE	RED OPAQUE MULTICOLORS	NONE	EMOTIONAL EXPERIENCE UNITY WITH ANOTHER	I BLEND
5TH HIGHER MIND	RESPONSIBILITY DIVINE WILL HOLY SPIRIT UNIVERSAL CONSCIOUSNESS	THOUGHT FOCUSING ACTION OF THOUGHT	COBALT BLUE AZURE BLUE PURPLE	VOICE WITHIN	AWARENESS STRENGTH HIGHER FORCE CONNECTION	I WILL
6TH CASUAL	WISDOM HIGHER SELF UNIVERSAL LOVE	PEACE, SECURITY	PRISMATIC PASTELS WITH GOLD AND WHITE LIGHT PINK, ELECTRIC BLUE, WHITE	WHITE NOISE	SPIRITUAL ECSTASY	I KNOW
7TH KETHERIC	BODY/SOUL MERGE LIFE FORCE HIGHER MIND SPIRITUAL STRENGTH	ENERGY SOURCE	GOLD	HUMMING	PEACE & SECURITY	I AM

AURAS ARE AN ATMOSPHERE ARISING FROM AND SURROUNDING THE BODY. COLORS VARY AND ARE CONSTANTLY CHANGING WITHIN THE AURIC FIELD.

BACH FLOWERS

A WHOLISTIC FLOWER REMEDY FOR EMOTIONAL PROBLEMS

PROBLEM TRAIT	EMOTIONAL PROBLEM	FLOWER NAME	RESULT
APPREHENSION	FEAR	ASPEN	FEARLESSNESS
EASILY DISCOURAGED	UNCERTAINTY	GENTIAN	PERSERVERANCE
ENVY, JEALOUSY	OVERSENSITIVITY	HOLLY	TOLERANCE
HARMFUL TO SELF AND OTHERS	FEAR	CHERRY PLUM	MENTAL CONTROL
HOPELESSNESS	UNCERTAINTY	GORSE	HOPE
INDIFFERENCE	LACK OF INTEREST	CLEMATIS	INTEREST
INTOLERANCE CRITICISM	OVERCARING	BEECH	TOLERANCE
MISGUIDED ACTIONS	UNCERTAINTY	CERATO	INTUITION
OVERWHELMED BY RESPONSIBILITY	DESPAIR	ELM	CONFIDENCE
PAST NOSTALGIA	LACK OF INTEREST	HONEYSUCKLE	LETTING GO
POSSESSIVENESS	OVERCARING	CHICKORY	SELFLESSNESS
REPETITIVE MISTAKES	LACK OF INTEREST	CHESTNUT BUD	KEEN OBSERVATION
SELF CONCERN	LONELINESS	HEATHER	SELFLESSNESS
SELF DISGUST	DESPAIR	CRAB APPLE	SELF SATISFIED
SUBSERVIENCE	OVERSENSITIVITY	CENTAURY	MAINTAINING ONE'S WILL
TORTURE BEHIND CHEERFULNESS	OVERSENSITIVITY	AGRIMONY	OPTIMISM

BACH FLOWERS

A WHOLISTIC FLOWER REMEDY FOR EMOTIONAL PROBLEMS

PROBLEM TRAIT	EMOTIONAL PROBLEM	FLOWER NAME	RESULT
APATHY	LACK OF INTEREST	WILD ROSE	INTEREST
COMPLETE EXHAUSTION	LACK OF INTEREST	OLIVE	PEACE OF MIND
DEEP GLOOM	LACK OF INTEREST	MUSTARD	SERENITY
DISLIKES CHANGE	OVERSENSITIVITY	WALNUT	ABILITY TO ADJUST
EXTREME ANGUISH	DESPAIR	SWEET CHESTNUT	OPTIMISM
EXTREME FEAR	FEAR	ROCK ROSE	HEROISM
GUILT	DESPAIR	PINE	BALANCED SENSE
IMPATIENCE	LONELINESS	IMPATIENS	UNDERSTANDING
OVERENTHUSIASM	OVERCARING	VERVAIN	CALMNESS
PRIDE	LONELINESS	WATER VIOLET	TRANQUILITY
PROCRASTINATION	UNCERTAINTY	HORNBEAM	FACE PROBLEMS
RESENTMENT	DESPAIR	WILLOW	CLEARS BODY & MIND TENSION
SAD ABOUT ILLNESS	DESPAIR	OAK	HOPE, COURAGE
SELF DENIAL	OVERCARING	ROCK WATER	EXPERIENCE ENJOYMENT
TRAUMA	DESPAIR	STAR OF BETHLEMHEM	RELIEF
VACILLATION	UNCERTAINTY	SCLERANTHUS	BALANCE

CABALA
TREE OF LIFE

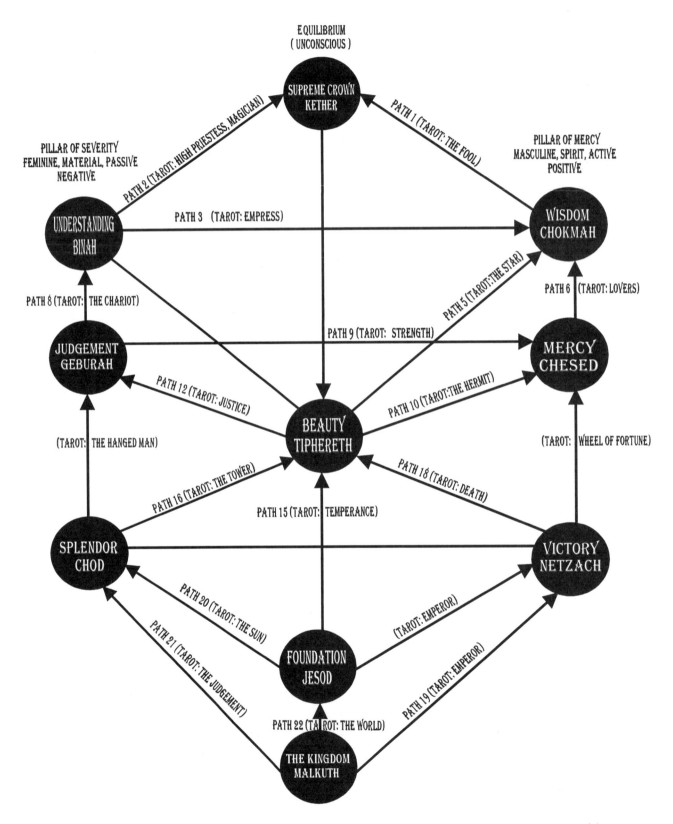

EQUILIBRIUM
(UNCONSCIOUS)

SUPREME CROWN
KETHER

PATH 1 (TAROT: THE FOOL)

PILLAR OF SEVERITY
FEMININE, MATERIAL, PASSIVE
NEGATIVE

PATH 2 (TAROT: HIGH PRIESTESS, MAGICIAN)

PILLAR OF MERCY
MASCULINE, SPIRIT, ACTIVE
POSITIVE

PATH 3   (TAROT: EMPRESS)

UNDERSTANDING
BINAH

WISDOM
CHOKMAH

PATH 8 (TAROT: THE CHARIOT)

PATH 5 (TAROT: THE STAR)

PATH 6   (TAROT: LOVERS)

PATH 9 (TAROT: STRENGTH)

JUDGEMENT
GEBURAH

MERCY
CHESED

PATH 12 (TAROT: JUSTICE)

PATH 10 (TAROT: THE HERMIT)

(TAROT: THE HANGED MAN)

BEAUTY
TIPHERETH

(TAROT: WHEEL OF FORTUNE)

PATH 18 (TAROT: DEATH)

PATH 16 (TAROT: THE TOWER)

PATH 15 (TAROT: TEMPERANCE)

SPLENDOR
CHOD

VICTORY
NETZACH

PATH 20 (TAROT: THE SUN)

(TAROT: EMPEROR)

PATH 21 (TAROT: THE JUDGEMENT)

FOUNDATION
JESOD

PATH 19 (TAROT: EMPEROR)

PATH 22 (TAROT: THE WORLD)

THE KINGDOM
MALKUTH

44

CABALA
TREE OF LIFE

SEPHIRA NAME	SOURCE	BODY PART	TRAIT	COLOR	PILLAR	PLANET
KETHER	SUPREME CROWN	HEAD	PRIMORDIAL FORCE	WHITE	EQUILIBRIUM	
TIPHERETH	BEAUTY	CHEST	UNIVERSAL AWARENESS	YELLOW	EQUILIBRIUM	SUN
JESOD	FOUNDATION	GENITALS	MATERIAL WORLD	PURPLE	EQUILIBRIUM	MOON
MALKUTH	THE KINGDOM	WHOLE BODY	PHYSICAL	BROWN	EQUILIBRIUM	
BINAH	UNDERSTANDING	HEART	INTELLIGENCE	BLACK	SEVERITY	SATURN
GEBURAH	JUDGEMENT	LEFT ARM	POWER	RED	SEVERITY	MARS
CHOD	SPLENDOR	LEFT LEG	GLORY	ORANGE	SEVERITY	MERCURY
CHOKMAH	WISDOM	BRAIN	ENLIGHTENMENT	SILVER	MERCY	
CHESED	MERCY	RIGHT ARM	GREATNESS LOVE, TRUTH	BLUE	MERCY	JUPITER
NETZACH	VICTORY	RIGHT LEG	ETERNAL FORM	GREEN	MERCY	VENUS

CARD FORTUNE TELLING

CARD	♥ MEANING	♣ MEANING	♦ MEANING	♠ MEANING
ACE	PLEASURE, JOY	TALENT, HIGH AMBITION	MONEY, CONSTRUCTIVE POWER	FORCE, POWER
KING	DEPENDABLE MAN OF GOOD WILL & INTEGRITY	RESERVED MAN OF DIVERSIFIED INTERESTS.	COMPLEX MAN WITH HIDDEN ASSETS	HONEST, INTELLIGENT, POWERFUL MAN
QUEEN	LOVE, JOY, A GOOD WOMAN	SHREWD WOMAN OF SOCIAL GRACES	PASSIONATE, WOMAN WITH SOCIAL PRESTIGE	PSYCHIC WOMAN WHO CONCEALS EMOTIONS
JACK	ROMANCE FRIENDSHIP	SINCERE, HONEST HARD WORKING YOUNG PERSON	CROSSROADS OF LIFE	IMMATURE YOUNG PERSON
10	GOOD NEWS, A MESSANGER	INEXPERIENCED YOUTH	ESCAPE FROM CONFINEMENT, JOURNEY	BARRIER, WALL, END OF DELUSION
9	HAPPINESS	SUCCESS, WORK SATISFACTION	GOOD WISH FULFILLED, BAD WISH REBOUNDED	UNPREDICTABLE CHANGES, CATASTROPHE
8	GIFT	BALANCE, HARMONY, QUIET DELIGHT	FINANCIAL/SPIRITUAL BALANCE	CONTENTMENT HAVEN
7	LOVER'S QUARREL	ILLUSIONARY SUCCESS	UNRESOLVED FINANCES DISTRESS	PARTIAL SUCCESS, DIVISION
6	ADVANCEMENT, STEP UP	SOCIAL LIFE OPPORTUNITY, GOOD FORTUNE	WELL BEING, ECONOMIC SECURITY	ANXIETY, SUSPENDED MOTION
5	DISAPPOINTMENT REGRET	AVOID QUARRELS WITH FRIENDS	CLASH OF WILLS	SEPERATION, REMORSE
4	HAPPINESS, OPPORTUNITY THROUGH WORK	STRENGTHENING OF FRIENDSHIP	SUCCESS BUSINESS FINANCE	HEALING, RECUPERATION
3	DISAPPOINTMENT IN LOVE	UNPLEASANT SOCIAL EPISODE	LEGAL DOCUMENT	SUDDEN RESOLUTION
2	LOVE LETTER, GOOD NEWS, UNEXPECTED PLEASURE	SOCIAL INVITATION	UNEXPECTED COMMUNICATION ABOUT MONEY, BUSINESS	MINOR STUBBLING BLOCK

CARD FORTUNE TELLING

15 CARD SPREAD

USE STANDARD PLAYING CARDS.
THINK OF A QUESTION.
SHUFFLE RYTHMICALLY.
CHOOSE CARDS AT ANY TIME AND
PROCEED TO LAY THEM OUT AS
THEY ARE SELECTED IN THE
FOLLOWING LAYOUT:

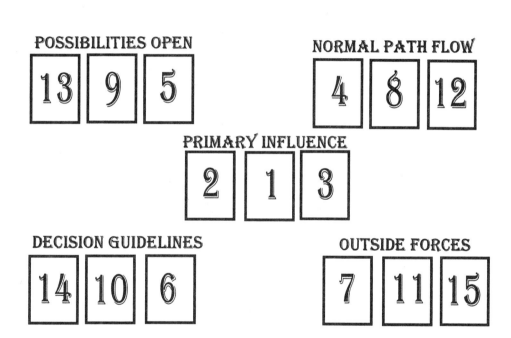

POSSIBILITIES OPEN

| 13 | 9 | 5 |

NORMAL PATH FLOW

| 4 | 8 | 12 |

PRIMARY INFLUENCE

| 2 | 1 | 3 |

DECISION GUIDELINES

| 14 | 10 | 6 |

OUTSIDE FORCES

| 7 | 11 | 15 |

CARD 1: QUERENT TRAIT OR PRIMARY LIFE INFLUENCE
CARD 2 & 3: QUERENT PERSONALITY OR SURROUNDING SITUATION
CARD 4, 8, 12: NORMAL LIFE PATH FLOW
CARD 13, 9, 5: ALTERNATE LIFE PATH; OPEN POSSIBILITITES
CARD 14, 10, 6: PRESENT/FUTURE DECISION MAKING GUIDELINES
CARD 7, 11, 15: OUTSIDE FORCES
EACH CARD'S MEANING IS SHADED BY THOSE AROUND IT

SAHASRARA   7TH CHAKRA

AJNA   6TH CHAKRA

VISHUDDA   5TH CHAKRA

ANAHATA   4TH CHAKRA

MANIPURA   3RD CHAKRA

SWADHISTHANA   2ND CHAKRA

MULADHARA   1ST CHAKRA

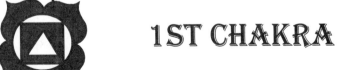

THE MAJOR CHAKRAS

THE ESOTERIC ENERGY CENTERS OF THE HUMAN BODY

CHAKRA	LOCATION	ATTRIBUTES	SPIRITUAL QUALITIES	PHYSIOLOGICAL/ ENDOCRINE	EXPERIENCE	COLOR	SOUND	INADEQUATE BALANCE RESULT
1ST ROOT COCCYGEAL MULADHARA	BASE OF SPINE	SURVIVAL INSTINCTS, REPRODUCTION, SEXUALITY, RAW CREATIVITY, VITALITY	INTUITIVE SELF PROTECTION	REPRODUCTIVE, GONADS	KINESTHETIC, TACTILE	RED WHITE	BUZZ	BLOOD DISORDERS INFERTILITY
2ND SACRAL SWADHISTHANA	SPLEEN OR NAVEL	EMOTIONS, MEMORY, ASSIMILATION	ACCESS TO KEY CHILDHOOD EXPERIENCES	GENITO-URINARY	EMOTIONAL	ORANGE VIOLET BLUE	EAR RINGING, RUNNING WATER	LUNG DISORDERS KIDNEY DISORDERS
3RD SOLAR PLEXUS MANIPURA	SOLAR PLEXUS	BALANCE INTELLECT PERSONAL POWER	PSYCHIC FEELING	DIGESTIVE / ADRENAL	GUT FEELING	GOLDEN YELLOW, PURPLE	FLUTE	STOMACH, LIVER PANCREAS
4TH HEART ANAHATA	CENTER OF CHEST	COMPASSION INNER HARMONY GROWTH	PSYCHIC HEALING	CIRCULATORY / THYMUS	UNCONDITIONAL LOVE	PINK GREEN	SINGING, BELLS, SEASHELL ROAR	HEART DISEASE HYPERTENSION
5TH THROAT VISHUDDA	HOLLOW OF THROAT	WILL, CREATIVITY DISCIPLINE SELF EXPRESSION	PSYCHIC HEARING	RESPIRATORY / THYROID	HEARING, SPEAKING	BLUE, TURQUOISE	WIND, OCEAN	THYROID LARNYX
6TH THIRD EYE AJNA	BETWEEN & SLIGHTLY ABOVE THE EYES	INTUITION, VISION IMAGINATION	PSYCHIC VISION	AUTONOMIC NERVOUS SYSTEM / PITUITARY	SIGHT OR VISION	INDIGO GREEN	OHM MANTRA	EYE DISORDERS
7TH CROWN SAHASRARA	VERY TOP OF THE HEAD	SPIRITUAL AWARENESS, UNIVERSAL MIND ACCESS	PROPHECY	CENTRAL NERVOUS SYSTEM / PINEAL	WHOLE CONCEPT	WHITE, PALE LAVENDER, VIOLET	SILENCE	NERVOUS DISORDERS MENTAL DISORDERS

CHEYENNE
MEDICINE WHEEL

RAISES AWARENESS, POWER & GROWTH EXPERIENCES

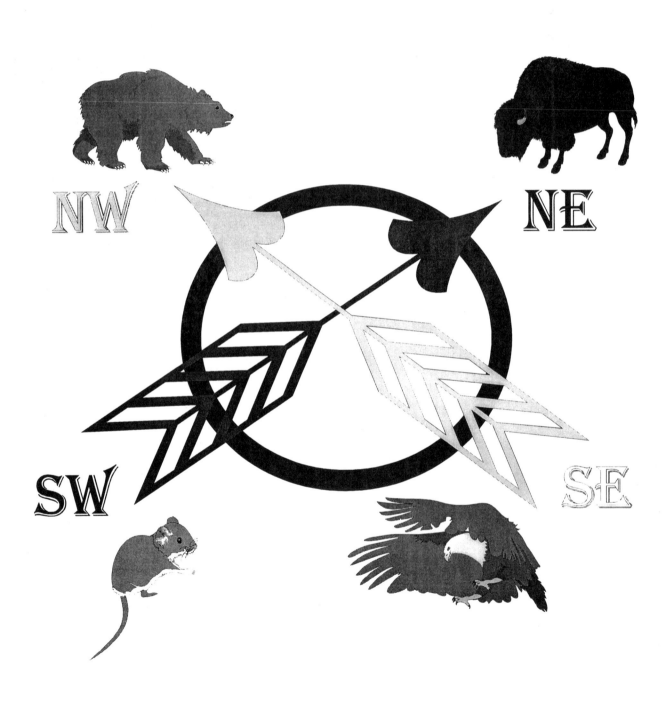

CHEYENNE
MEDICINE WHEEL

DIRECTION	COLOR	HOUSE	ELEMENT	ABODE	SOURCE
NORTHEAST	BLACK	BUFFALO		DOG SOLDIERS	POWER, DEATH, WISDOM, DISEASE, SILENCE
EAST	YELLOW BLUE		AIR	MEN'S LODGE	PAST MENTAL
SOUTHEAST	WHITE	EAGLE		PEACE CHIEFS	LIGHT, LIFE, RENEWAL, ILLUMINATION
SOUTH	RED GREEN		FIRE	WAR CHIEFS	PRESENT PHYSICAL
SOUTHWEST	RED	MOUSE		SINGERS STORYTELLERS MEDIUMS HEALERS	GROWTH, WEATHER, INNOCENCE
WEST	BLACK BROWN		WATER	WOMEN'S LODGE	FUTURE EMOTIONAL
NORTHWEST	YELLOW	BEAR		COUNCIL LODGE	HARVEST, INTROSPECTION, PERFECTION
NORTH	PURPLE SKY BLUE		EARTH	HUNTERS GATHERERS	SPIRITUAL TRANSFORMATION

CHINESE ELEMENTS

ELEMENT	SEASON	DIRECTION	RELATION	PLANET	COLOR	ANIMAL	KEY WORDS
WATER	WINTER	NORTH	DEATH	MERCURY	BLACK	TORTOISE	INTELLIGENCE CHANGE COMMUNICATION
FIRE	SUMMER	SOUTH	INITIATION	MARS	RED	PHOENIX	ENERGY STIMULATION
WOOD	SPRING	EAST	BIRTH	JUPITER	GREEN	DRAGON	INNOVATION CREATIVITY
METAL	AUTUMN	WEST	REPOSE	VENUS	WHITE	TIGER	VALOR BUSINESS CONFLICT
EARTH		CENTER	LOVE	SATURN	YELLOW	DRAGON	STABILITY

CHINESE ELEMENTS

ELEMENT	BODY PART	ACCUPRESSURE MERIDIANS	QUALITIES	ENERGY ATTRIBUTES	REGULATES
WATER	KIDNEYS BLADDER	KIDNEY BLADDER	REST RELAXATION	STORES ENERGY RESERVES	BODY FLUIDS BONES, HEARING, MEMORY
FIRE	HEART PERICARDIUM	SMALL INTESTINES TRIPLE WARMER	WELL BEING SELF ESTEEM	ENERGY PRESENCE	BLOOD CIRCULATION EMOTIONAL SYSTEM
WOOD	GALL BLADDER	LIVER	INNER VISION CREATIVITY	DISTRIBUTES ENERGY	ANGER
METAL	LARGE INTESTINES LUNGS	LARGE INTESTINES LUNGS	MATERIAL & SPIRITUAL NEEDS	RELEASES UNNECESSARY ENERGY	BREATHING, EMOTIONAL BALANCE
EARTH	STOMACH	SPLEEN	BALANCE PERSPECTIVE	BALANCES PHYSICAL & EMOTIONAL ENERGY	COMPASSION, SEXUAL DISFUNCTION, DIGESTION

CHINESE HERBS

NAME	PART USED	USED FOR
ACONITE FU TZU	ROOT	SEXUAL POTENCY, FLATULENCE, PAIN, ARTHRITIS, NUMBNESS, EXCESS MOISTURE
APRICOT SEED KU XING REN	KERNEL	LUNGS, LARGE INTESTINES
ASTRAGALUS HUANG CHI	ROOT	INCREASE ENERGY, DIURETIC, SPLEEN, KIDNEYS, BUILD IMMUNE SYSTEM, BLOOD
BUPLEURUM CH'AI HU	ROOT	LIVER, DIZZINESS, ANXIETY, MUSCLE TONE
CHRYSANTHEMUM CHU HUA	FLOWERS	DIZZINESS, FEVER, HEADACHES, BLOOD, EYES, LIVER
CITRUS PEEL CHEN PI	PEEL	INDIGESTION, DIARRHEA, VOMITING, COLDS, ABDOMINAL PAIN, ENERGY CIRCULATION
DEER ANTLER LU RONG	CROSS SECTION OF ANTLER	HORMONE SYSTEM, APHRODISIAC
DONG QUAI	ROOT	MENUSTRATION, CRAMPS, ANEMIA, INSOMNIA, CONSTIPATION, INSOMNIA
DON SEN TANG SHEN	ROOT	INCREASES ENERGY, PANCREAS, SPLEEN, INFECTION, DIABETES, INFLAMMATION
ELEUTHERO	ROOT LEAVES	INSOMNIA, BRONCHITIS, HEART DISEASE, LOWER CHOLESTEROL & BLOOD PRESSURE
EPHEDRA MA HUANG	STEMS BRANCHES	CONGESTION, COUGHS, FLU, FEVERS, ASTHMA, ADRENALS
FU LING	WHOLE FUNGUS	DIURETIC, EMOTIONAL IMBALANCE, LUNG CONGESTION, INSOMNIA, SPLEEN, STOMACH
GELATIN	HIDES OF BLACK DONKEYS	BLOOD, HORMONES, LIVER
GINSENG JEN SHENG	ROOT	WHOLE BODY, HEART, BLOOD PRESSURE, CIRCULATION, INFLAMMATION, FEVER
HONEYSUCKLE YIN HUA	FLOWERS	DETOXIFIER, POISON IVY, RASHES, FLU

CHINESE HERBS

NAME	PART USED	USED FOR
HO SHOU WU FO TI	ROOT	ENERGY, STRENGTH, FERTILITY, DIABETES, LIVER, KIDNEYS, BLOOD, HYPOGLYCEMIA
JUJUBE DATE DA T'SAO	WHOLE DATE	ENERGY, FORGETFULLNESS, DIZZINESS, INSOMNIA, STOMACH, SPLEEN, PANCREAS
LICORICE GAN T'SAO	ROOT	WHOLE BODY, ADRENAL, ULCERS, COLDS, FLU, LIVER, BLOOD DETOXIFIER
LONGAN BERRIES LONG YEN ROU	BERRIES	WOMEN'S REPRODUCTIVE ORGANS, ANEMIA, FORGETFULLNESS, HEART, PANCREAS
LYCII GAY GEE	BERRIES	FEVERS, BRONCHITIS, KIDNEYS, LIVER, COLDS, CLOUDY VISION, BLOOD PURIFIER
PAI SHU	ROOT	DIURETIC, INDIGESTION, DIARRHEA, EDEMA, STOMACH, PANCREAS, KIDNEYS
PEONY SHAO-YAO	ROOT	LIVER, SKIN ERUPTIONS, INFECTIONS, CRAMPS, UTERUS, ANEMIA
PLATYCODON JIE GENG	ROOT	LUNGS, SORE THROAT, ASTHMA, BRONCHITIS, PNEUMONIA
PUERARIA KUZU ROOT	ROOT	GASTROINTESTINAL, COLDS, FLU
REHMANNIA SOK DAY-SANG DAY	ROOT	BLOOD PURIFIER, BONES, TENDONS, ANEMIA, WEAK HEART, FATIGUE, KIDNEYS
SALVIA DANG SHEN	ROOT	MENSES REGULATION, BLOOD TONIC, ITCH, ABODMINAL EXTENSION, RHEUMATISM
SCUTELLARIA HUANG CHI	ROOT	NERVES, LARGE INTESTINES, HEART, GALL BLADDER, LIVER, LUNGS
SILERIS FANG-FENG	ROOT	CHILLS, JOINT PAIN, HEADACHE, NUMBNESS, FLU, TETANUS
TIENCHI	ROOT	HEMORRAGE, HEART, CIRCULATION, FATIGUE, STRESS, WOUNDS, STOMACH
WILD GINGER XI XIN	ROOT	ENERGY, CONGESTION, SPASMS

CHINESE HOROSCOPE

Years of the Rat	Years of the Ox	Years of the Tiger	Years of the Rabbit
1/31/00 - 2/18/01	2/19/01 - 2/07/02	2/08/02 - 1/28/03	1/29/03 - 2/15/04
2/18/12 - 2/05/13	2/06/13 - 1/25/14	1/26/14 - 2/13/15	2/14/15 - 2/02/16
2/05/24 - 1/23/25	1/24/25 - 2/12/26	2/13/26 - 2/01/27	2/02/27 - 1/22/28
1/24/36 - 2/10/37	2/11/37 - 1/30/38	1/31/38 - 2/18/39	2/19/39 - 2/07/40
2/10/48 - 1/28/49	1/29/49 - 2/16/50	2/17/50 - 2/05/51	2/06/51 - 1/26/52
1/28/60 - 2/14/61	2/15/61 - 2/04/62	2/05/62 - 1/24/63	1/25/63 - 2/12/64
2/15/72 - 2/02/73	2/03/73 - 1/22/74	1/23/74 - 2/10/75	2/11/75 - 1/30/76
2/02/84 - 2/19/85	2/20/85 - 2/08/86	2/09/86 - 1/28/87	1/29/87 - 2/16/88
2/19/96 - 2/06/97	2/07/97 - 1/27/98	1/28/98 - 2/15/99	2/16/99 -2/4/2000

Year of the Dragon	Years of the Snake	Years of the Horse	Years of the Goat
2/16/04 - 2/03/05	2/04/05 - 1/24/06	1/25/06 - 2/12/07	2/13/07 - 2/01/08
2/03/16 - 1/22/17	1/23/17 - 2/10/18	2/11/18 - 1/31/19	2/01/19 - 2/19/20
1/23/28 - 2/09/29	2/10/29 - 1/29/30	1/30/30 - 2/16/31	2/17/31 - 2/05/32
2/08/40 - 1/26/41	1/27/41 - 2/14/42	2/15/42 - 2/04/43	2/05/43 - 1/24/44
1/27/52 - 2/13/53	2/14/53 - 2/02/54	2/03/54 - 1/23/55	1/24/55 - 2/11/56
2/13/64 - 2/01/65	2/02/65 - 1/20/66	1/21/66 - 2/08/67	2/09/67 - 1/29/68
1/31/76 - 2/17/77	2/18/77 - 2/06/78	2/07/78 - 1/27/79	1/28/79 - 2/15/80
2/17/88 - 2/05/89	2/06/89 -1/26/90	1/27/90 - 2/14/91	2/15/91 - 2/03/92

Year of the Monkey	Years of the Rooster	Years of the Dog	Years of the Pig
2/02/08 - 1/21/09	1/22/09 - 2/09/10	2/10/10 - 1/29/11	1/30/11 - 2/17/12
2/20/20 - 2/07/21	2/08/21 - 1/27/22	1/28/22 - 2/15/23	2/16/23 - 2/04/24
2/06/32 - 1/25/33	2/26/33 - 2/13/34	2/14/34 - 2/03/35	2/04/35 - 1/23/36
1/25/44 - 2/12/45	2/13/45 - 2/01/46	2/02/46 - 1/21/47	1/22/47 - 2/09/48
2/12/56 - 2/17/57	1/31/57 - 2/17/58	2/18/58 - 2/07/59	2/08/59 - 1/27/60
1/30/68 - 2/16/69	2/17/69 - 2/05/70	2/06/70 - 1/26/71	1/27/71 - 2/14/72
2/16/80 - 2/04/81	2/05/81 - 1/24/82	1/25/82 - 2/12/83	2/13/83 - 2/01/84
2/04/92 - 1/22/93	1/23/93 - 2/09/94	2/10/94 - 1/30/95	1/31/95 - 2/18/96

CHINESE HOROSCOPE

SIGN	FRIENDSHIP	OPPOSITE	LOVE/MARRIAGE	PERSONALITY
RAT	OX	HORSE	DRAGON, OX MONKEY	INTELLIGENCE, CHARM, CLEVER, HUMOUROUS
OX/ BUFFALO	RAT	GOAT	SNAKE, RAT ROOSTER	TRADITIONAL, HONEST, STEADFAST, PATIENT
TIGER	RABBIT	MONKEY	HORSE DRAGON	LEADER, EXTROVERT, ROMANTIC, IMPULSIVE
RABBIT	TIGER	ROOSTER	GOAT PIG	INSIGHT, DECISIVE INDEPENDENT, HEALER
DRAGON	SNAKE	DOG	RAT MONKEY	ELEGANT, FORTUNATE, GRANDEUR, IMAGINATIVE
SNAKE	DRAGON	PIG	OX ROOSTER	MYSTIC, ATTRACTIVE, SUBTLE, ELEGANT
HORSE	GOAT	RAT	GOAT, DOG, TIGER	INTELLIGENT, FREE, SOCIABLE, HUMOROUS
GOAT	HORSE	OX	PIG RABBIT	DEMOCRACTIC, ARTISTIC, AFFECTIONATE, GENTLE
MONKEY	ROOSTER	TIGER	RAT DRAGON	CLEVER, VERSATILE, BOLD, INTELLIGENT
ROOSTER	MONKEY	RABBIT	SNAKE, OX DRAGON	ROMANTIC, GENEROUS, DETERMINED, HONEST
DOG	PIG	DRAGON	TIGER HORSE	STEADFAST, FRIENDLY, PROTECTIVE, LOYAL
PIG/ BOAR	DOG	SNAKE	GOAT RABBIT	DOMESTIC, TRANQUIL, SINCERE, HONEST

FAVORITE COLORS

PERSONAL COLOR	PERSONALITY TRAITS
RED	OUTGOING, ASSERTIVE, VITALITY, IMPULSIVE, SEXUAL ENERGY, LOVING NATURE, OPTIMISTIC, COMPLAINER
ORANGE	GOOD NATURED, FRIENDLY, LOYAL, CHARITABLE, SWAYED BY OUTSIDE OPINIONS, PEOPLE ORIENTED
YELLOW	IMAGINATIVE, INTELLIGENT, ALOOF, LONER, SHY, GOOD FRIEND, NEED TO HELP THE WORLD, NERVOUS ENERGY
GREEN	SOCIAL, UPFRONT, COMPETITIVE, REPUTABLE, MORAL, GOOD CITIZEN, FAMILY ORIENTED, BALANCED
BLUE	INTROSPECTIVE, SOBER, SENSITIVE, DELIBERATE, CONSERVATIVE, ANNOYED BY STUPIDITY, DEVOTED
PURPLE	INTELLIGENT, SPIRITUAL, WITTY, OBSERVANT, VERBOSE, ARTISTIC, VAIN, CREATIVE
BROWN	CONSCIENTIOUS, DEPENDABLE, STEADFAST, SHREWD, OBSTINATE, SENSUAL, DOWN TO EARTH
GREY	CAUTIOUS, CONSERVATIVE, COMPOSED, PEACEFUL, AGREEABLE, INDEPENDENT
BLACK	WORLDLY, POLITE, CONVENTIONAL, REGAL, DIGNIFIED, RECEPTIVE, ABOVE AVERAGE

COLOR

COLOR	ASPECT	QUALITIES	CHAKRA	SEPHIRAH	MUSICAL NOTE
WHITE	UNIVERSAL ENERGY PEACE	DIVINITY, SPIRIT, PROTECTION, CLEANSING	7TH CROWN	THE CROWN KETHER	C, B
GOLD	LIFE FORCE SPIRITUAL STRENGTH	SPIRITUAL VITALITY, SUBSTANCE	3RD & 7TH SOLAR, CROWN		D
SILVER	COMMUNICATION ENLIGHTENMENT	SPIRITUAL TRUTH	CORD OF 7TH CROWN	WISDOM CHOKMAH	G SHARP A FLAT
MAGENTA	INTUITION INSPIRATION	CREATIVE, VITALITY	6TH, 7TH 3RD EYE, CROWN		B
PURPLE	QUEST SPIRITUALITY	SPIRITUAL GROWTH, ESTEEM	6TH, 7TH 3RD EYE, CROWN	FOUNDATION JESOD	B
INDIGO	VISION INNOVATION	INVENTION, CLARITY, INSIGHT	6TH 3RD EYE		B
BLUE	TRUTH TRANQUILITY	HEALING, DEVOTION, SPIRITUAL TRANQUILITY	5TH, 6TH THROAT, 3RD EYE	MERCY CHESED	A, A SHARP B FLAT
TURQUOISE	CREATIVITY THOUGHT	IDEALISM, DISCIPLINE, ARTISTIC CREATION	5TH THROAT		G
GREEN	LOVE HEALING	GROWTH, BALANCE ABUNDANCE	4TH HEART	VICTORY NETZACH	F, F SHARP G FLAT
YELLOW	PRECISION VISION	CLARITY, CENTERED, INTELLIGENCE	3RD SOLAR	BEAUTY TIPHERETH	E, D SHARP E FLAT
ORANGE	COURAGE ESTEEM	BRAVERY, PRIDE, AMBITION	2ND SPLEEN	GLORY CHOD	C SHARP
RED	ENERGY PASSION	LOVING NATURE, VITALITY, SEXUAL ENERGY	1ST BASE	JUDGEMENT GEBURAH	C
PINK	BEAUTY EMOTIONAL HARMONY	JOY, TENDERNESS, COMPASSION	4TH HEART		F, F SHARP G FLAT
BROWN	EARTHINESS SENSUALITY	PRACTICALITY, SENSUAL AWARENESS		THE KINGDOM MALKUTH	
BLACK	RECEPTIVITY VOID	STATE OF GRACE, POSSIBILITY, CREATIVE VOID		UNDERSTANDING BINAH	

HEALING COLORS

Studies using spectral colors have shown some success in aiding the healing process. Our emotional and physical state may change when special colored lights are used on the body.

COLOR	ACTIVATES:	USED FOR:	
RED	SENSORY NERVOUS SYSTEM BLOOD CIRCULATION SYMPATHETIC NERVOUS SYSTEM LEFT CEREBRAL BRAIN	ANEMIA ASTHMA BRONCHITIS CONSTIPATION	LISTLESSNESS PARALYSIS PNEMONIA ENDOCRINE TROUBLE
YELLOW	MOTOR NERVES MUSCLE ENERGY NERVE REGENERATION LYMPHATIC SYSTEM	ARTHRITIS CONSTIPATION DIABETES DIGESTION	ECZEMA LIVER DISEASE KIDNEY DISEASE MENTAL DEPRESSION
ORANGE	THYROID GLAND PULSE RATE SPLEEN PANCREAS	ASTHMA COLDS GALL STONES PMS	RESPIRATORY DISEASE RHEUMATISM TUMORS MENTAL EXHAUSTION
GREEN	MUSCLE & BONE GROWTH EMOTIONAL STABILIZATION TISSUE GROWTH TENSION RELIEF	INSOMNIA EXHAUSTION ULCERS LARYNGITIS	HEART PROBLEMS BACK PROBLEMS VENERAL DISEASE NERVOUS DISORDERS
BLUE	METABOLISM BLOODSTREAM BALANCE MIND RELAXATION VITALITY	BALDNESS BURNS ULCERS VOMITING	SKIN DISEASE TOOTH INFECTION EYE INFLAMMATION GASTROINTESTINAL
INDIGO	PARATHYROID BLOOD PURIFICATION MUSCLE TONE HEMOSTATIC AGENT	APPENDICITIS DEAFNESS PNEUMONIA EAR DISEASE	MENTAL ILLNESS NASAL DISEASE EYE DISEASE THROAT DISEASE
VIOLET	SPLEEN UPPER BRAIN BONES IONIC POTASSIUM/SODIUM BALANCE	CONCUSSION BONE GROWTH SCIATICA TUMORS	BLADDER PROBLEMS NEURALGIA ABDOMINAL CRAMPS NERVOUS DISORDERS

HEALING COLORS & MUSIC

Each color is associated with a musical note. Color produces physical vibrations to the eye and music produces sound vibrations to the ears. It is said that by applying the appropriate musical sound and color vibrations we can change our emotional state and aid in healing ourselves.

COLOR	QUALITY	MUSICAL NOTE	PYTHAGOREAN QUALITY	VIBRATIONS PER SECOND
DEEP RED	SPIRITUAL ILLUMINATION	G	POSITIVE FORCE LIFTING GRATITUDE	384
RED ORANGE	THE ABSOLUTE CREATIVE FORCE	A	HEALTH DESTRUCTION	213
YELLOW	WILL POWER UNITY UNDERSTANDING	B	PLANT & ANIMAL DENSE VIBRATION PENETRATION	240
YELLOW GREEN	LOVE CHASTITY	C	PURIFICATION	256
GREEN BLUE	SPIRIT RENEWAL	D	VITALITY	288
BLUE VIOLET	HEALING CLEANSING	E	HARMONY HEALING	320
VIOLET	SPIRITUAL POWER	F	PURIFICATION VISUALIZATION	341

CRYSTALS, GEMSTONES, METALS & ORES

NAME	COLOR	SPIRITUAL ATTRIBUTES	HEALING PROPERTIES	ENERGY
AGATE	VARIEGATED	INCREASES ACCEPTANCE	UPSET STOMACH	SOUL/BODY HARMONY
AMETHYST	PALE VIOLET TO DEEP PURPLE	PLANETARY WELL BEING SPIRITUAL AWARENESS	INSOMNIA, WORRY, ASTHMA, ALLERGIES, BLOOD PURIFIER, SMOG PROTECTION	RECHARGES THE BODY BALANCES THE MIND CALMS THE EMOTIONS
AQUAMARINE	LIGHT BLUE TO DEEP GREEN	SPIRITUAL AWARENESS MEDITATION AID	THYMUS GLAND	PEACE
AZURITE	AZURE TO DARK BLUE	KIND & PATIENT LOVE CLEANSING & PURIFYING	SPLEEN	COMFORT
BLOODSTONE	DEEP GREEN WITH SPLOTCHES OF RED	POWERFUL	SPINE	COMING TOGETHER OF HIGHER SELF
CARNELIAN	RED TO ORANGE	CURIOSITY STIMULANT	LIVER, REMOVES LETHARGY	ENERGY FOCUS
CHALCEDONY	GRAY, WHITE BLUE, BLACK	MAINTAINS POSITIVE VIBRATIONS	WOUNDS	PROTECTION REPEL NEGATIVE ENERGY
CHRYSOPHASE	GREEN	SPIRTULIST'S INSULATOR	BODY/MIND CLEANSING	PROTECTION
CHRYSOBERYL	YELLOW TO GREEN	CHARITY	ADRENAL GLANDS EMOTIONAL PROBLEMS	LOVE, GENEROSITY, FORGIVENESS
CITRINE	YELLOW	SUPPORT OF WILL	BODY ENERGY	SELF DISCIPLINE
CRYSTAL QUARTZ	CLEAR	SPIRITUAL AWARENESS CLEARNESS	ANY ILLNESS	BENEFITS MIND, BODY, SOUL
	ROSE	JOY & SELF LOVE	DEPRESSION	RIDS EMOTIONAL PAIN
DIAMOND	WHITE	INFINITY	CHEMICAL IMBALANCE	PROTECTION SOUL ENERGY
EMERALD	DEEP GREEN	CLEAR CONSCIENCE LOVE, WISDOM	EYES, DIABETES	HEALING, WISDOM PROSPERITY
FLUORITE	GREEN, WHITE PURPLE	VISIONARY INSIGHT	MECHANICAL RADIATION	ONENESS
GARNET	GREEN, TO BROWN YELLOW RED	CONTEMPLATION IDENTIFY PAST LIFE	HEART, BLOOD, PITUITARY	CREATIVE ENERGY BALANCE, PEACE
JADE	GREEN	DREAM WORK ENHANCER TRANQUILITY, PEACE	HEART, KIDNEYS, SPLEEN, HAIR	REACHES PROBLEM DEPTH, HARMONY
	LAVENDAR		MENTAL PROBLEMS	LOVE, SECURITY
	RED		EMOTIONAL PROBLEMS	ANSWERS PROBLEMS
	ORANGE		LACK OF ENERGY	ERADICATES APATHY
	YELLOW		POOR DIGESTION	SOOTHING
	BLUE		MENTAL THOUGHTS	PEACE
JASPER	RED, GREEN, YELLOW, BLUE	HELPS LONG TERM CHANGES	GENERAL BODY	SUPPLEMENT BODY ENERGY
KUNZITE	PALE PINK LILAC	AIDS DISCIPLINE	BLOOD FLOW	FOUNDATION

CRYSTALS, GEMSTONES, METALS & ORES

NAME	COLOR	SPIRITUAL ATTRIBUTES	HEALING PROPERTIES	ENERGY
LAPIS LAZULI	DEEP BLUE	PROMOTES CLAIRVOYANCE	MEMORY, EYESIGHT	CALMS THE MIND
MALACHITE	LIGHT TO DARK GREEN	HEART & SOUL CONSCIOUSNESS	EMOTIONAL BLOCKS	AMPLIFIES POSITIVE & NEGATIVE QUALITIES
MOONSTONE	MILKY BLUE OPALESENCE	REFLECTION OF INNER SELF INTUITVENESS	HEART, BLOOD, CIRCULATORY	EMOTIONAL BALANCE
ONYX	BLACK	INTUITIVENESS TO OTHERS	INFECTION	STABILIZING/STRENGTHENING MIND & BODY
OPAL	WHITE REFRACTS ALL COLORS	AMPLIFIES PERSON'S OWN TRAITS	PURIFY BLOOD, VISION DISORDERS	SHOULD BE WORN BY BALANCED PERSON ONLY
PEARL	WHITE, YELLOW BLACK	AMPLIFIES PERSON'S TRAITS	SOFTENS EMOTIONS	PEACE OF MIND
PERIDOT	LIGHT GREEN	SEEING CLEARLY DISSOLVES PROBLEMS	SPIRIT HEALING	SOOTHING
PRISM	CLEAR	UNFOLDS INNER BEAUTY	MENTAL DISORDERS	CLARITY
RHODONITE	BLACK WITH PINK & YELLOW	COMPASSION	UPPER RESPIRATORY	COMPASSION
RUBY	DEEP RED	LOVE, TRUTH	BLOOD PURIFIER	BALANCES SEXUAL ENERGY
SAPPHIRE	BLACK, BLUE WHITE, GREY	LIGHTNESS, INTUITION	MIND & SPIRIT	JOY, SOOTHES MIND & SPIRIT
SARDONYX	BANDED RED & WHITE	DEFENSE	BONE MARROW	INCREASE DESIRE FOR CAUSES
TIGERS EYE	GOLDEN BROWN	ALL SEEING	MIND STRENGTH	SOUL VIBRATION WITH THE UNIVERSE
TOPAZ	GOLDEN YELLOW PALE BLUE, PINKISH BROWN	PROMOTES CONFIDENCE	NEUROLOGICAL DISORDERS	LIGHT, JOY, LOVE PHYSICAL STRENGTH STAMINA
TOURMALINE	BLACK	PROTECTS FROM NEGATIVE INFLUENCES	INTESTINAL TRACT	GROUNDING
	BLUE	CLEAR COMMUNICATION	THROAT	COMMUNICATION
	GREEN	SPIRITUALITY ACCEPTANCE GREATER CONSCIOUSNESS	FEVERS	ABILITY TO LOVE, PROSPERITY
	PINK	EASES EXPRESSIONS OF LOVE TO OTHERS	EMOTIONAL PAIN	ENTHUSIAM, JOY
TURQUOISE	SKY BLUE, APPLE GREEN	WISDOM	TENSION IN JAW, MOUTH & THROAT	STRENGTH, VITALITY
ZIRCON	RED, BROWN, GREEN YELLOW, LIGHT BLUE	PEACE WITHIN ONESELF	LUNGS, BREATHING	HEALING OF SPIRIT
CINNABAR	BRICK RED	EVALUATION	SOLAR PLEXUS, HEART	POSITIVE ENERGY
COPPER	COPPER	ELIMINATES METALLIC WASTE IN BODY	BODY IMPURITIES	CLEANSING
GALENA	SILVER GREY	RECEPTIVITY	MENTAL DISORDERS	FEELING/THOUGHT RECEPTIVITY
GOLD	GOLD	POSITIVE VIBRATIONS	BODY ENERGY	INCREASES ENERGY
LODESTONE	GREY	UNIVERSAL THOUGHT	LUNGS	NEW IDEAS
SILVER	SILVER	MIND CLARITY	STRESS	STRENGTH

DICE FORTUNETELLING

CIRCLE TOSS METHOD FOR QUESTIONS

DRAW A 12 INCH DIAMETER CIRCLE.
THINK OF YOUR QUESTION.
USE THREE DIE AND TOSS WITHIN THE CIRCLE.
ADD ALL THE NUMBERS ON DICE TOGETHER
AND LOOK UP NUMBERED MEANING BELOW.

NOTES:
NO DICE THROWING FRIDAYS & SUNDAYS.
IF DICE LANDS OUTSIDE CIRCLE IT IS UNLUCKY.
IF ALL DICE LAND OUTSIDE CIRCLE, RETOSS.
IF ALL DICE LAND OUTSIDE AGAIN, STOP.

VALUE	MEANING	VALUE	MEANING
3	UNEXPECTED GOOD NEWS. A GIFT.	11	UNHAPPINESS.
4	DISAPPOINTMENT. BAD LUCK.	12	GOOD NEWS.
5	WISH FULFILLED.	13	GRIEF. WORRY.
6	FINANCIAL LOSS. DISHONEST FRIEND OR LOVED ONE.	14	NEW FRIEND OR ADMIRER.
7	SETBACKS. GUARD YOUR SECRETS.	15	CAUTION. AVOID ARGUMENTS.
8	STRONG OUTSIDE FORCES.	16	A GOOD JOURNEY.
9	LUCK IN LOVE. RECONCILIATION.	17	CHANGE.
10	DOMESTIC HAPPINESS. BUSINESS PROMOTION.	18	SUCCESS, ADVANCEMENT, HAPPINESS, WEALTH

DICE FORTUNE TELLING

CIRCLE TOSS METHOD FOR FUTURE REVELATIONS

DRAW A 12 INCH DIAMETER CIRCLE.
DIVIDE CIRCLE INTO 12 EQUAL SEGMENTS.
WRITE THE FOLOWING LETTERS, 1 PER SEGMENT.
  A, B, C, D, E, F, G, H, I, J, K, L
SHAKE & TOSS 3 DIE INTO THE CIRCLE.

READ THE NUMBERED MEANING BELOW FROM THE
NUMBER OF EACH DIE PER THE SEGMENT IT'S IN.

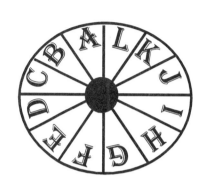

SEGMENT	MEANING
A	NEXT YEAR
B	FINANCES
C	TRAVEL
D	DOMESTIC AFFAIRS
E	PRESENT
F	HEALTH
G	LOVE & MARRIAGE
H	LEGAL MATTERS
I	PRESENT EMOTIONAL STATE
J	CAREER
K	FRIENDS
L	ENEMIES

NUMBER	MEANING
1	FAVORABLE RELATE TO OTHER DICE.
2	SUCCESS DEPENDS ON FRIENDS.
3	EXCELLENT FOR SUCCESS.
4	DISAPPOINTMENT. DIFFICULTIES.
5	GOOD FORTUNE
6	UNCERTAINTY

DOMINOES FORTUNE TELLING

DOMINO	MEANING	DOMINO	MEANING
SIX/SIX	HAPPINESS, SUCCESS, PROSPERITY IN ALL	FOUR/THREE	HAPPINESS, SUCCESS
SIX/FIVE	PATIENCE AND TENACITY	FOUR/TWO	SETBACK OR LOSS. BEWARE DECEITFUL FRIEND
SIX/FOUR	QUARREL UNSUCCESSFUL LAW SUIT	FOUR/ONE	FINANCIAL PROBLEMS, PAY DEBTS
SIX/THREE	TRAVEL, ENJOYMENT, A GIFT	FOUR/BLANK	DISAPPOINTMENT, BAD NEWS
SIX/TWO	GOOD LUCK FOR AN HONEST PERSON	THREE/THREE	WEDDING, GOOD FINANCES
SIX/ONE	WEDDING, END TO A PROBLEM	THREE/TWO	GOOD CHANGE, CAUTION WITH MONEY
SIX/BLANK	BEWARE OF A FALSE FRIEND	THREE/ONE	ANSWER IS NO, UNEXPECTED USEFUL NEWS
FIVE/FIVE	CHANGE BRINGS SUCCESS	THREE/BLANK	UNEXPECTED PROBLEMS
FIVE/FOUR	FINANCIAL LUCK BUT AVOID INVESTING NOW	TWO/TWO	SUCCESS & HAPPINESS
FIVE/THREE	SERENITY, GOOD NEWS	TWO/ONE	LOSS OF PROPERTY OR MONEY, HAPPY SOCIAL LIFE
FIVE/TWO	BIRTH, SOCIABILITY, ENJOYMMENT	TWO/BLANK	TRAVEL & NEW FRIENDS
FIVE/ONE	NEW LOVE AFFAIR OR ENDING AN OLD LOVE AFFAIR	ONE/ONE	PLEASURE & HARMONY, MAKE DECISION
FIVE/BLANK	SADNESS	ONE/BLANK	BE CAREFUL
FOUR/FOUR	HAPPINESS, CELEBRATION	BLANK/BLANK	NEGATIVE ASPECTS ALL AREAS

DOMINOES FORTUNE TELLING

METHOD:
1. THINK OF A QUESTION.
2. SHUFFLE DOMINOES FACE DOWN.
3. CHOOSE 1ST DOMINO, READ MEANING ON BACK.
4. RETURN DOMINO TO PILE, RESHUFFLE.
5. SELECT 2ND DOMINO, REPEAT STEP 4.
6. SELECT 3RD AND LAST DOMINO, READ MEANING.

NOTE: IF SAME TILE IS DRAWN TWICE, WISH WILL BE GRANTED SOON. OLD LEGEND SAYS ONLY 1 WISH PER SITTING AND ONLY 1 SITTING PER WEEK.

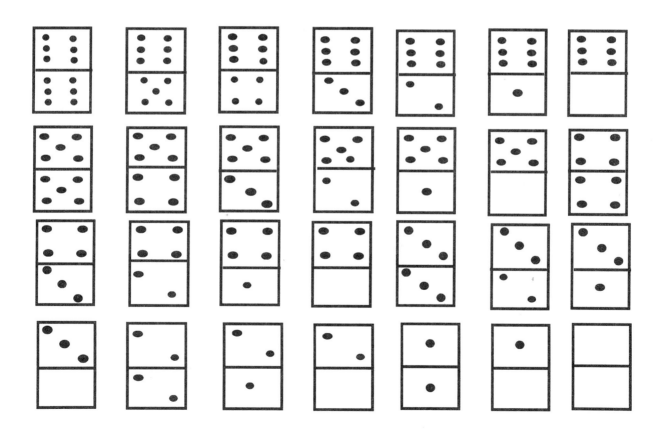

GODS

NAME	ORIGIN	DESCRIPTION	NAME	ORIGIN	DESCRIPTION
AANI	EGYPT	DOG HEADED APE	DAGAN	BABYLON	EARTH
ABU (AKU)	BABYLON	SKY, SUN	DAGDA	CELTIC	CHIEF
ADAD (ADDA)	BABYLON	WIND, STORM	DEVA (DEWA)	HINDU	DIVINE BEING
AEGIR	NORSE	SEA	DIS	GREEK/ROMAN	UNDERWORLD
AESCULAPIUS	GREEK/ROMAN	MEDICINE	DYAUS	HINDU	HEAVEN
AGNI	HINDU	FIRE	DYLAN	WELSH	CHIEF
AKAL	HINDU	IMMORTAL	EA (HEA,ENKI)	BABYLON	CHIEF
AMEN	EGYPT	KING	ER	NORSE	WAR
AMON	EGYPT	KING, SUN	EROS	GREEK	LOVE
AMOR	ROMAN	LOVE	ETANA	BABYLON	EAGLE RIDER
ANAT	ASSYRIAN	SKY	EURUS	GREEK	SOUTHEAST WIND
APOLLO	GREEK	SUN, PROPHECY, MUSIC	FAUN	ROMAN	HERDS, HALF GOAT
APSU (ASSUR)	BABYLON	CHAOS	FREY	NORSE	FERTILITY
ARES	GREEK	WAR	GWYTH	CYMRIC	SOLAR
ASUN	ASSYRIAN	WAR	HADES	GREEK	UNDERWORLD
BABBAR	BABYLON	SUN	HELIOS	GREEK	SUN
BACCHUS	ROMAN	WINE	HERMES	GREEK	HERALD
BALDER	NORSE	LIGHT	HORUS	EGYPT	HAWK HEADED
BEL	BABYLON	CHIEF	HOTH	NORSE	BLIND GOD
BES	EGYPT	EVIL, PLEASURE	INTI	INCAN	SUN
BRAGI	NORSE	POETRY	IRA	BABYLON	WAR
CIVA (SIVA)	HINDU	SUPREME	JOVE	ROMAN	CHIEF GOD
COMUS	GREEK/ROMAN	MIRTH, REVELRY, JOY	KA	HINDU	GOD OF UNKNOWN
CRONUS	GREEK	TITAN	KAMA	HINDU	LOVE
CUPID	ROMAN	LOVE	KEB (GEB)	EGYPT	EARTH

GODS

NAME	ORIGIN	DESCRIPTION	NAME	ORIGIN	DESCRIPTION
KRISHNA	HINDU	AVATAR OF VISHNU	RAMA	HINDU	VISHNU
LER	CELTIC	SEA	SET (SETH)	EGYPT	EVIL
LOK (LOKI)	NORSE	DISCORD, MISCHIEF	SHAMASH	BABYLON	SUN
LUGH	CELTIC	LIGHT, SUN	SIN (ENZU)	BABYLON	MOON
MARS	ROMAN	WAR	SIRIS	BABYLON	ALCOHOL
MENT	EGYPT	FALCON HEADED	SOBK	EGYPT	CROCODILE HEAD
MIN	EGYPT	PROCREATION	SOL	ROMAN	SUN
MOMUS	GREEK	RIDICULE	SU	EGYPT	SOLAR
MORS	ROMAN	DEATH	TEM	EGYPT	SUN
NABU (NEBU)	BABYLON	WISDOM	THOR	NORSE	THUNDER
NEPTUNE	ROMAN	SEA	THOTH	EGYPT	WISDOM, MAGIC
NEREUS	GREEK	SEA	TRITON	GREEK	SEA
ODIN	NORSE	CHIEF GOD, WISDOM	TY	NORSE	SKY, WAR
ORCUS	ROMAN	DEAD	UTUG	BABYLON	SUN
OSIRIS	EGYPT	UNDERWORLD	VAN	NORSE	SEA
PAN	GREEK	FLOCKS, FOREST	VAYU	HINDU	WIND
PLUTO	GREEK	UNDERWORLD	VISHNU	HINDU	SUPREME
PLUTUS	GREEK	WEALTH	VULCAN	ROMAN	FIRE
POSEIDON	GREEK	SEA	YAMA	HINDU	JUDGE OF THE DEAD
PTAH	EGYPT	MEMPHIS	ZEUS	GREEK	OLYMPIA, GOD HEAD
RA	EGYPT	SUN	ZIO	NORSE	SKY

GREAT GODDESS
CIRCLE OF POWER

RAISES POWER, AWARENESS & GROWTH EXPERIENCES

DIRECTION	RELATION	ELEMENT	TIME	COLOR	ANIMAL	TOOL	POWER
EAST	MIND	AIR	DAWN	WHITE VIOLET	EAGLE	SWORD	TO KNOW
SOUTH	SPIRIT	FIRE	NOON	RED ORANGE	LION	WAND	TO DO
WEST	FEELING	WATER	DUSK	SEA GREEN BLUE/GREY PURPLE	FISH	CUP	TO DARE
NORTH	MYSTERY	EARTH	MID-NIGHT	BROWN BLACK	BULL	PENTACLE	TO LISTEN

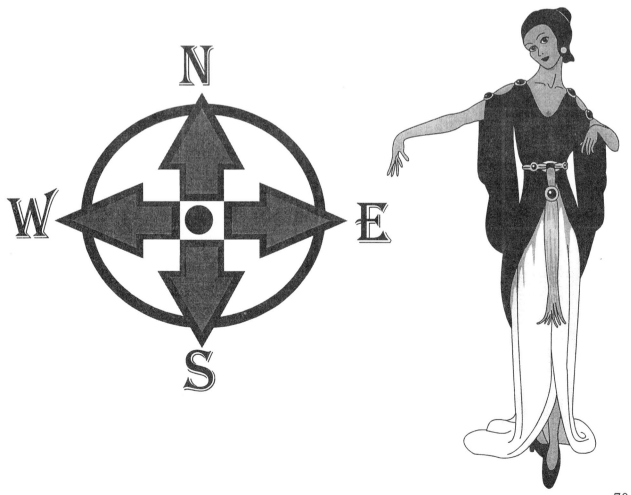

GODDESS SYMBOLS

SYMBOL	MEANING
AMPHIBIAN	REGENERATION
BEAR	BIRTH GIVER
BEE	REGENERATION
BIRD	GIVER OF ALL
BULL	SOURCE OF LIFE
BUTTERFLY	REGENERATION
CIRCLE	DIVINE ENERGY CENTER
CRESCENT	ENERGY
DOE	MOTHER

SYMBOL	MEANING
WHITE DOG	DEATH
DOVE	SOUL
DUCK	LUCK, WEALTH
EGG	REGENERATION
LETTER M	LIFE GIVER
OWL	DEATH MESSENGER
RAM	MAGIC
SNAKE	LIFE SOURCE
SOW	SACRED ANIMAL EARTH MOTHER

GODDESSES

NAME	ORIGIN	DESCRIPTION	NAME	ORIGIN	DESCRIPTION
AI (AYA)	BABYLON	SHAMASH CONSORT	EIR	GREEK/ NORSE	HEALING
ANA (ANU)	CELTIC	MOTHER, QUEEN	EOS	GREEK	DAWN
ANTA (APET)	EGYPT	MATERNITY	EPONA	ROMAN	HORSES
APHRODITE	GREEK	LOVE	ERDA	NORSE	EARTH
ARA	GREEK	DESTRUCTION	ERIS	GREEK	DISCORD
ARTEMIS	GREEK	MOON, NATURE	ERUA	BABYLON	MOTHER
ASTARTE	PHOENICIAN	LOVE, FERTILITY	FLORA	ROMAN	FLOWERS
ATE	GREEK	DISCORD, MISCHIEF	FREYA	NORSE	LOVE, BEAUTY
ATHENA	GREEK	WISDOM	GE (GAIA)	GREEK	EARTH MOTHER
ATROPOS	GREEK	THREAD CUTTER	HATHOR	EGYPT	LOVE, MIRTH
AURORA	ROMAN	DAWN	HECATE	GREEK	MOON, MAGIC
BAST	EGYPT	CAT HEADED	HEL	NORSE	UNDERWORLD
BUTO	EGYPT	SERPENT	HERA	GREEK	QUEEN
CERES	ROMAN	EARTH	IRIS	ROMAN	RAINBOW
CHLORIS	GREEK	FLOWERS	ISIS	EGYPT	COW HEADED
CLOTHO	GREEK	THREAD SPINNER	ISHTAR	BABYLON	CHIEF, LOVE
CYBELE	GREEK	NATURE	JUNO	ROMAN	QUEEN
DEMETER	GREEK	AGRICULTURE	KALI	HINDU	EVIL
DEVI	HINDU	DIVINITY	LACHESIS	GREEK	THREAD LENGTH
DIANA	ROMAN	MOON, HUNT	LUNA	ROMAN	MOON
DON	BRYTHONIC	GOD'S ANCESTOR	MAAT (MA, MUT)	EGYPT	TRUTH, JUSTICE

GODDESSES

NAME	ORIGIN	DESCRIPTION	NAME	ORIGIN	DESCRIPTION
MATRIS	BABYLON	MOTHERS	RHEA	GREEK	MOTHER OF GODS
MINERVA	CELTIC	WISDOM	SALUS	ROMAN	PROSPERITY
MOIRA	EGYPT	FATE	SATI	EGYPT	QUEEN
MORN	GREEK	FATE	SELENA	GREEK	MOON
NANAI	BABYLON	ANU'S DAUGHTER	SPES	ROMAN	HOPE
NANNA	NORSE	FLOWERS	SRI (LAKSHMI)	HINDU	BEAUTY, LUCK
NEMISIS	GREEK	REVENGE	TERRA	ROMAN	EARTH
NIKE	GREEK	VICTORY	UMA	HINDU	SPLENDOR
NINA	BABYLON	WATERY DEEP	URD	NORSE	DESTINY
NONA	ROMAN	FATE	USAS	HINDU	DAWN
NOX	ROMAN	NIGHT	VAC	HINDU	SPEECH
NUT	EGYPT	HEAVEN	VENUS	ROMAN	LOVE
OPS	ROMAN	HARVEST	VESTA	ROMAN	HEARTH
RAN	NORSE	SEA	VOR	NORSE	BETROTHAL

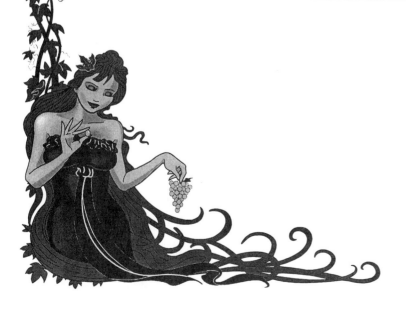

HERBS

HERB/USE	HERB/USE	HERB/USE	HERB/USE
ACORN/TB, AIDS	BUCHU/PMS	CORIANDER/ANTISEPTIC	GINKGO/ALZHEIMER'S
AGRIMONY/ASTRINGENT	BUCKTHORN/LAXATIVE	CRANBERRY/URINARY INFECTION	GINSENG/IMMUNE SYSTEM
ALOE/BURNS,POISON IVY	BURDOCK/FOOD POISONING	DAMANIA/DEPRESSION	GOLDENSEAL/COLITIS
ANGELICA/ARTHRITIS	CALENDULA/EAR ACHES	DANDELION/STOMACH	GOTU KOLA/IMMUNE SYSTEM
ANISE/MENOPAUSE	CARAWAY/DIGESTION	DILL/ABDOMINAL PAIN	GRAVELROOT/URINARY
ASAFETIDA/GAS, CANDIDA	CASCARA/CONSTIPATION	DUSTY MILLER/CLOUDY VISION	HAWTHORNE/HEART DISEASE
BALM/ANXIETY, INSOMNIA	CATNIP/ANXIETY	ECHINACEA/ARTHRITIS	HOP/INSOMNIA
BARBERRY/ BRONCHITIS	CELERY SEED/STRESS	ELECAMPANE/RESPIRATORY	HOREHOUND/COUGH
BASIL/IMMUNE SYSTEM	CHAMOMILE/DIGESTION	EPHEDRA/HAY FEVER	HORSETAIL/ANTI-INFLAMMATORY
BAY/ANXIETY	CHAPPARAL/CANCER	EUCALYPTUS/ANTISEPTIC	HYSSOP/COLDS, FLU
BAYBERRY/COLDS, FLU	CINNAMON/ANESTHETIC	EVENING PRIMROSE/PMS	IRISH MOSS/DRY COUGH
BLACKBERRY/FEVERS	CLOVE/PARASITIC	FENNEL/DIGESTION AID	JUNIPER/GOUT, GAS
BLACK COHOSH/NERVES	COCOA/JET LAG	FENUGREEK/ HIGH CHOLESTEROL	KAVA KAVA/FATIGUE
BLACK HAW/MENOPAUSE	COFFEE/DECONGESTANT	FEVERFEW/HEADACHE	KELP/ANTISEPTIC
BLOODROOT/SKIN CANCER	COLTSFOOT/COUGHS	GARLIC/ANTIBIOTIC	KOLA/FATIGUE
BLUE COHOSH/MENSTRUAL	COMFREY/HEALING	GENTIAN/ARTHRITIS	LARKSPUR/LICE
BONESET/COLDS, FLU	CORN SILK/URINARY INFECTIONS	GINGER/MOTION SICKNESS	LAVENDER/ANTIDEPRESSANT

HERBS

HERB/USE	HERB/USE	HERB/USE	HERB/USE
LEMON BALM/TENSION	MUELLIN/LYMPH CONGESTION	RHUBARB/CONSTIPATION	THYME/COUGHS
LICORICE/SORE THROAT	MYRRH/PAIN, GAS	ROSEMARY/JOINT INFLAMMATION	TURMERIC/ANTISEPTIC
LINDEN FLOWER/HYPERTENSION	NETTLE/ANEMIA, WEAKNESS	RUE/CRAMPS, SPASMS	UVA URSI/HERPES
LOBELIA/ASTHMA	OAK BARK/DYSENTERY	SAFFRON/HIGH CHOLESTEROL	VALERIAN/INSOMNIA
LOQUAT/HICCOUGHS	OATS/DEPRESSION	SAGE/FOOD POISONING	VERVAIN/LIVER DISORDERS
MARJORAM/DIGESTION	OREGANO/DIGESTION AID	SARSAPARILLA/VD	VIOLET/SORE THROAT
MARSH MALLOW/COLDS	PAPAYA/DIGESTION	SASSAFRAS/ARTHRITIS	WALNUT/STRENGTH
MATE/STIMULANT	PARSLEY/DIURETIC BREATH FRESHNER	SAVORY/COUGH	WILD CHERRY/ULCERS
MAY APPLE/WARTS	PAU D'ARCO/CHRONIC FATIGUE	SAW PALMETTO/PROSTRATE	WILD YAM/GALL STONES
MEADOWSWEET/PAIN	PASSIONFLOWER/INSOMNIA	SENNA/CONSTIPATION	WILLOW/ANALGESIC
MILK THISTLE/HEPATITIS	PENNYROYAL/NERVOUS TENSION	SHEPERD'S PURSE/BLEEDING	WITCH HAZEL/DISCHARGE
MINTS/ANTIBIOTIC	PLANTAIN/ANTI-INFAMMATORY	SKULLCAP/NERVOUSNESS	WOOD BETONY/ANXIETY
MISTLETOE/IMMUNE SYSTEM	POPPY/PAIN, ANXIETY	SLIPPERY ELM/ULCERS	WORMWOOD/HEPATITIS
MOTHERWORT/CIRCULATION	PSYLLIUM/CONSTIPATION	SUMA/ENERGY TONIC	YARROW/HEMORRHOIDS
MUGWORT/LIVER PROBLEMS	RASBERRY/MENSTRUAL	STJOHN'S WORT/AIDS	YELLOW DOCK/ANEMIA
MUIRA-PUAMA/IMPOTENCE	RED CLOVER/CANCER	TARRAGON/ANTISEPTIC	YERBA SANTA/RESPIRATORY
MULBERRY/ADRENALS	RED PEPPER/HEADACHE	TEA/HIGH CHOLESTEROL	YUCCA/ARTHRITIS

I CHING FORTUNE

HEXAGRAM COIN TOSS METHOD

WRITE YOUR QUESTION. THINK OF YOUR QUESTION AND TOSS 3 COINS 6 TIMES. FIRST TOSS REPRESENTS 6TH LINE, SECOND 5TH LINE, ETC. DRAW THE CORRESPONDING LINE FROM THE COIN TABLE FOR EACH TOSS. THEN GO TO TABLE BELOW AND FIND THE HEXAGRAM NUMBER. READ THE CORRESPONDING NUMBERED MESSAGE ON REVERSE SIDE. A DOT REPRESENTS A CHANGING LINE. CREATE A REVERSE HEXAGRAM & READ BOTH HEXAGRAM MEANINGS.

Coin Table

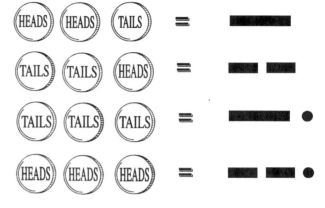

Example Reverse Hexagram

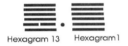

Hexagram 13   Hexagram 1

EXAMPLE: CH'IEN LOWER TRIGRAM **AND** K'AN UPPER TRIGRAM = **HEXAGRAM 5**

Toss 6, Line 1
Toss 5, Line 2
Toss 4, Line 3
Toss 3, Line 4
Toss 2, Line 5
Toss 1, Line 6

UPPER TRIGRAM → / LOWER TRIGRAM ↓	CH'IEN	CHEN	K'AN	KEN	K'UN	SUN	LI	TUI
CH'IEN	1	34	5	26	11	9	14	43
CHEN	25	51	3	27	24	42	21	17
K'AN	6	40	29	4	7	59	64	47
KEN	33	62	39	52	15	53	56	31
K'UN	12	16	8	23	2	20	35	45
SUN	44	32	48	18	46	57	50	28
LI	13	55	63	22	36	37	30	49
TUI	10	54	60	41	19	61	38	58

I CHING FORTUNE

HEXAGRAM	MEANING	HEXAGRAM	MEANING	HEXAGRAM	MEANING	HEXAGRAM	MEANING
1	CREATIVE POWER	17	ADAPTING	33	RETREAT	49	CHANGING
2	NATURAL RESPONSE	18	REPAIR	34	GREAT POWER	50	COSMIC ORDER
3	DIFFICULT BEGINNINGS	19	PROMOTION	35	PROGRESS	51	SHOCKING
4	INEXPERIENCE	20	CONTEMPLATING	36	CENSORSHIP	52	MEDITATION
5	CALCULATED WAITING	21	REFORM	37	FAMILY	53	DEVELOPING
6	CONFLICT	22	GRACE	38	CONTRADICTION	54	SUBORDINATE
7	COLLECTIVE FORCE	23	DETERIORATION	39	OBSTACLES	55	ZENITH
8	UNITY	24	REPEATING	40	LIBERATION	56	TRAVELING
9	RESTRAINED	25	INNOCENCE	41	DECLINE	57	PENETRATING INFLUENCE
10	CONDUCT	26	POTENTIAL ENERGY	42	BENEFIT	58	ENCOURAGING
11	PROSPERING	27	NOURISHING	43	RESOLUTION	59	REUNITING
12	STAGNATION	28	CRITICAL MASS	44	TEMPTATION	60	LIMITATIONS
13	COMMUNITY	29	DANGER	45	ASSEMBLING	61	INSIGHT
14	SOVERIGNITY	30	SYNERGY	46	ADVANCEMENT	62	CONSCIENTIOUSNESS
15	MODERATION	31	ATTRACTION	47	ADVERSITY	63	AFTER THE END
16	HARMONIZE	32	CONTINUING	48	THE SOURCE	64	BEFORE THE END

I CHING TRIGRAMS

NAME	TRIGRAM	DIRECTION/ANIMAL	EMBLEM/ELEMENT	TIME OF DAY/YEAR	BODY PART	QUALITIES
CH'IEN		NORTHWEST/DRAGON, HORSE	HEAVEN/METAL	DAYTIME/EARLY WINTER	HEAD	CREATIVE VITALITY STRENGTH
CHEN		EAST/FLYING DRAGON	THUNDER/WOOD	EARLY MORNING/SPRING	FOOT	ACTIVITY GROWTH AROUSING
K"AN		NORTH/PIG	WATER, MOON/WATER	MIDNIGHT/MID WINTER	EAR	MENTAL DIFFICULT MYSTERIOUS
KEN		NORTHEAST/DOG, RAT BIRDS	MOUNTAIN/WOOD	DAWN/LATE WINTER	HAND	CALM STILL WAITING
K'UN		SOUTHWEST/MARE, OX	EARTH/EARTH	NIGHT/EARLY AUTUMN	BELLY	RECEPTIVE ADAPTABLE NOURISHING
SUN		SOUTHEAST/HEN	WIND/WOOD	MID MORNING/EARLY SUMMER	THIGH	HONEST GROWTH GENTLE
LI		SOUTH/TOAD, CRAB, SNAIL	LIGHTENING/FIRE	NOON/MID SUMMER	EYE	INTELLIGENT CONSCIOUS ILLUMINATING
TUI		WEST/SHEEP	LAKE/WATER. METAL	TWILIGHT/LATE AUTUMN	MOUTH	PLEASURE REFLECTION SATISFACTION

I CHING
TRIGRAMS

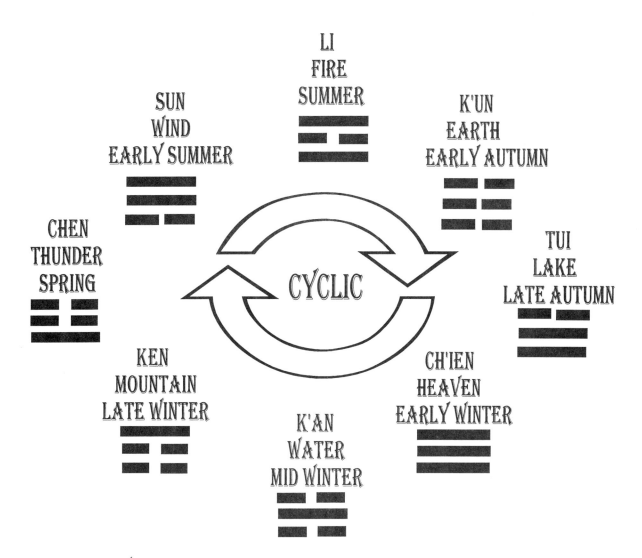

KING WEN TRIGRAM ARRANGEMENT

▬ ▬ YIN - PASSIVE/YIELDING
▬▬▬ YANG - STRONG/ACTIVE

NATIVE AMERICAN
ANIMAL SPIRIT COMMUNICATION

According to tradition if an animal crosses your path it has a meaning.

ANIMAL/MEANING	ANIMAL/MEANING	ANIMAL/MEANING	ANIMAL/MEANING
ANTELOPE/ACTION	COCKROACH/SURVIVAL	HAWK/OPPORTUNITY	PELICAN/SAVER
ARMADILLO/DEFENDED	COW/DOCILE	HERON/SPIRITUAL	PIG/INTELLIGENCE
BADGER/AGGRESSIVE	COYOTE/CUNNING	HORSE/FREEDOM	PORCUPINE/PROTECTION
BAT/MACABRE	CRICKET/DISHARMONY	HUMMINGBIRD/JOY	POSSUM/AVOIDANCE
BEAR/STRENGTH	CROW/PORTENT	LARK/WEATHER	QUAIL/FAMILY
BEAVER/RESOURCEFUL	DEER/LOVELINESS	LIZARD/OLD WISDOM	RABBIT/GENTLE
BEETLE/HIDDEN KNOWLEDGE	DOG/LOYALTY	LYNX/PSYCHIC	RACCOON/ENTERPRISING
BIGHORN SHEEP/CONQUEROR	DONKEY/HELPFUL	MAGPIE/KNOWLEDGE	RAT/SURVIVAL
BULL/SEXUAL ENERGY	DOLPHIN/UNIVERSAL MIND	MEADOWLARK/PROTECTION	SEA GULL/FREEDOM
BUFFALO/ABUNDANCE	DUCK(WILD)/ADVENTURE	MOLE/TRUST	SKUNK/DEFENSE
BUTTERFLY/FRIENDLY	EAGLE/SPIRIT MESSANGER	MOUSE/BUSY	SNAKE/RAW ENERGY
CANARY/JOY	ELK/BRAVE	MOUNTAIN LION/LEADER	SPIDER/FATE
CARDINAL/BEAUTY	FLAMINGO/GRACE	MULE/STUBBORN	SQUIRREL/RESOURCEFUL
CAT/INDEPENDENT	FLY/PARASITIC	OWL/DIVINER	TURKEY/FORGETFUL
CHICKADEE/OPTIMISM	FOX/WILY	OTTER/PLAYFUL	WHALE/CONSCIOUSNESS
CHICKEN/FOOLISH	FROG/SORCERY	PHEASANT/GUISE	WOLF/ORGANIZE
CHAMELEON/ADAPTABLE	GOOSE (SNOW)/FIDELITY (DOMESTIC)/QUARRELSOME	PIGEON(IN AIR)/MISSION (ON GROUND)/INERTIA	WOODPECKER/RESOURCEFUL

NATIVE AMERICAN ANIMAL DREAM SPIRITS

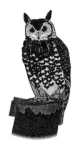

According to tradition when you see an animal in your dreams it has a meaning.

ANIMAL	MEANING	ANIMAL	MEANING
BADGER	SOMEONE IS PUSHING YOU, YOU ARE NOT FIGHTING BACK.	HARE	BE AWARE OF BEAUTY AROUND YOU.
BEAR	USE YOUR POWER AND HELP.	HORSE	TAKE RISKS. PERSONAL FREEDOM SUPPRESSED.
BEAVER	GET BUSY & COMPLETE PROJECT.	MOUSE	TENDENCY TO TALK, NO INSIGHT.
BUFFALO	DEVELOP LEADERSHIP QUALITIES.	OWL	TREMENDOUS UNDEVELOPED PSYCHIC POTENTIAL.
COYOTE	PUT MORE FUN IN YOUR LIFE.	RACCOON	GET ORGANIZED. HAVE MORE FUN.
CROW	GET HELP TO DISCOVER BETRAYAL.	RAM	SEEK SPIRITUAL NOT MATERIAL PLEASURES.
DEER	NEED FOR BEAUTY AND GENTLENESS.	SEA GULL	GET OUT OF OLD PATTERN.
DOLPHIN/ WHALE	COMMUNITY CONCERNS.	SKUNK	NEED FOR PROTECTION AND DEFENSE.
EAGLE/ HAWK	GROWTH AND IMPORTANT LESSONS.	SNAKE	USE YOUR WISDOM AND INTELLIGENCE.
ELK/ MOOSE	NEED TO BALANCE MALE/FEMALE ENERGY. CONTACT OPPOSITE SEX.	SONGBIRD	MISSING ARTISTIC BEAUTY IN YOUR LIFE.
FROG	EXPAND YOUR SPIRITUALITY.	TURTLE	SLOW DOWN AND BE PATIENT.
FOX	BE MORE CUNNING.	WOLF	NEGLECTING FAMILY NEEDS.

NUMEROLOGY

1	2	3	4	5	6	7	8	9
A	B	C	D	E	F	G	H	I
J	K	L	M	N	O	P	Q	R
S	T	U	V	W	X	Y	Z	

LIFE CYCLE NUMBER: YOUR NAME*

BALANCE NUMBER: YOUR MONOGRAM (INITIALS)**

DESTINY NUMBER: YOUR BIRTHDATE**

To determine your life cycle number add the numeric values together.
e.g. L i n d a S m i t h
      3+9+5+4+1   1+4+9+2+8 = 46
      4+6 = 10
       1+0 = 1
 * Use the name you are best known by.
** Modifies your Life Cycle Number.

NUMEROLOGY

#	SYMBOL	PLANET	CYCLES	QUALITIES	LOVE / MARRIAGE	VOCATION	MONEY
1	○, 🌹 CIRCLE, ROSE	SUN	JAN 1 - FEB 9 NEW BEGINNIGS	PIONEERS, INNOVATORS, VISION, BENEVOLENCE, OUTGOING, PROTECTOR UNCHANGING, CREATIVE	BEST: 2, 6 OTHERS: 3, 4, 5. 7	ARTIST, BUSINESS, SCIENTIST, EDUCATOR, ENGINEER, PRODUCER, ADMINISTRATOR	RISK TAKERS
2	☯ YIN/YANG	MOON	FEB 10 - MAR 21 SEEKING KNOWLEDGE	COOPERATOR, SENSITIVE, IMAGINATIVE, HELPFUL, DIPLOMATIC, GENTLE, CONSTANT, DEVOTED, EVER CHANGING	BEST: 2, 4, 6 OTHERS: 1, 8, 3. 5	ACTORS, MIUSICIANS, MARRIAGE COUNSELOR, TEACHER, RESEARCH, ACCOUNTANT, NURSES	SECURE INVESTOR
3	△ TRIANGLE	JUPITER	MAR 22 - APR 30 SELF EXPRESSION	INTELLECTUAL, WITTY, GREGARIOUS, POPULAR, TALENTED, AFFECTIONATE, FRIENDLY, COMMUNITY	BEST: 1, 3, 5, 8 OTHERS: 2, 4, 6, 7, 9	WRITER, ENTERTAINER, PHOTOGRAPHER, PUBLISHING, ADVERTISING, ENGINEER, PUBLIC RELATIONS	EASY COME, EASY GO
4	✝, △ CROSS, PYRAMID	SATURN	MAY 1 - JUN 10 MAKING DECISIONS	JUSTICE, RESPONSIBLE, DEPENDABLE, SACRIFICE, INDIVIDUALIST, TOLERANT, GENIOUS, STUBBORN	BEST: 4, 7, 9 OTHERS: 2, 6, 1, 8	ENGINEERS, CONTRACTORS, JUDGES, MATHEMATICIAN, LAWYER, CRAFTSMEN, CHEMISTS, PHARMACISTS	PRUDENT, THRIFTY
5	⬠ PENTAGRAM	MERCURY	JUN 11 - JUL 21 NEW PLEASURES	INTELLIGENT, ADAPTABLE, SENSUOUS, IMPULSIVE, VERSATILE, DYNAMIC, BOLD, DECISIVE, ENTHUSIASTIC	BEST: 5, 3, 6 OTHERS: 7, 8	WRITERS, JOURNALISTS, ARTISTS, CRIMINAL LAW, AVIATORS, STOCK BROKERS, PUBLIC RELATIONS, ANY FIELD	GENEROUS, CASUAL
6	✡ STAR OF DAVID	VENUS	JUL 22 - AUG 31 INCREASED AWARENESS	HARMONIOUS, BEAUTIFUL, BALANCED, COMPASSIONATE, TEAM PLAYER, COURTEOUS, ROMANTIC, PRIDEFUL	BEST: 6, 2 OTHERS: 3, 5, 4	TEACHERS, DOCTORS, SOCIAL/WELFARE WORKERS, NURSES, BOOKKEEPERS, ACCOUNTANTS	SECURITY
7	🌈 RAINBOW	URANUS	SEP 1 - OCT 10 SOLITUDE & MEDITATION	INTELLIGENT, INTUITIVE, INDIVIDUALIST, MYSTERIOUS, PHILOSOPHER, SPIRITUAL, RECEPTIVE	BEST: 9, 4, 7 OTHERS: 3, 5, 1, 8	SCIENTIST, EDUCATOR, ARTIST, RELIGION, AGENTS, WRITERS, NAVIGATORS	ECONOMY
8	∞ FIGURE 8	MARS	OCT 11 - NOV 20 OVERCOMING OBSTACLES	STRENGTH, SUCCESSFUL, DETERMINED, POWERFUL, LOYAL, SELF DISCIPLINED, AMBITIOUS, PATIENT	BEST: 2, 7, 4, 9 OTHERS: 3, 5, 6, 2	EXECUTIVES, PLANNERS, BUSINESS, AUTHORITY FIGURE IN ANY FIELD	WELL TO DO, FLAIR
9	♎ ALPHA & OMEGA	NEPTUNE	NOV 21 - DEC 31 SERVICE TO MANKIND	LOVE FOR FELLOW MAN, NOBLE, PHILOSOPHER, LEADER, MYSTICAL, INSPIRATIONALIST	BEST: 4, 7, 9 OTHERS: 3, 6, 8	DOCTOR, SOCIAL WORKER, LECTURER, HYPNOTIST, LAW, TEACHER, ADVERTISING, FINANCE, RELIGIOUS LEADER	GENEROUS, BASIC

PALM READING

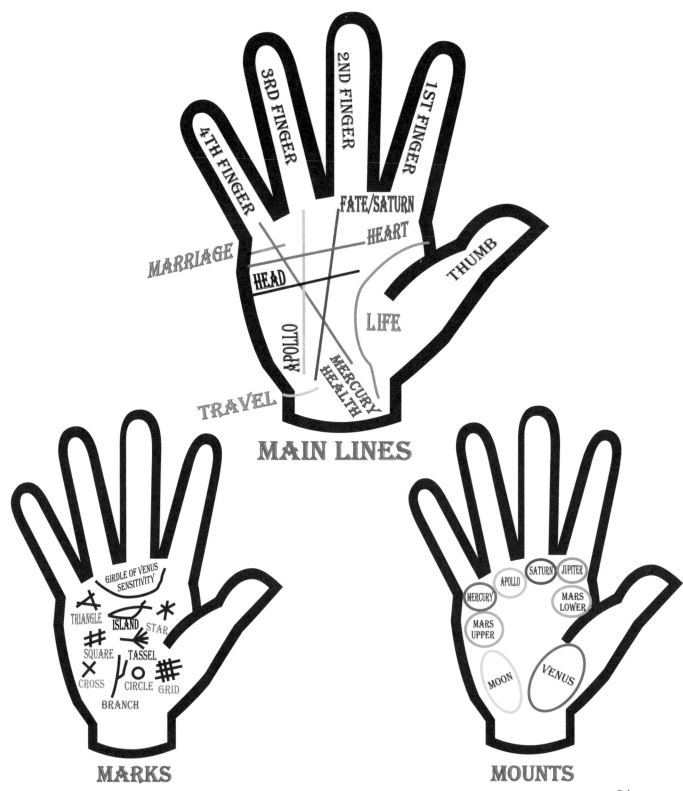

MAIN LINES

4TH FINGER · 3RD FINGER · 2ND FINGER · 1ST FINGER

FATE/SATURN

HEART

MARRIAGE

HEAD

THUMB

APOLLO

LIFE

MERCURY HEALTH

TRAVEL

MARKS

GIRDLE OF VENUS SENSITIVITY

TRIANGLE · STAR

ISLAND

SQUARE · TASSEL

CROSS · CIRCLE · GRID

BRANCH

MOUNTS

SATURN · JUPITER

APOLLO

MERCURY · MARS LOWER

MARS UPPER

MOON · VENUS

PALM READING

LEFT HAND - NATURAL TENDENCIES - RIGHT HAND - DEALS WITH LIFE

HAND TYPE / MEANING		HAND TYPE / MEANING	
BROAD & SQUARE	TRADITIONAL	BROAD	PRACTICAL
FLARED	ORIGINAL THINKER	LONG & NARROW	PSYCHIC, REFLECTIVE
LONG & BONY	PHILOSOPHICAL	MIXED	VERSATILE

MAIN LINES / ATTRIBUTES		MOUNTS / ATTRIBUTES	
HEAD	INTELLECT, REASONING	MERCURY	COMMUNICATION, WIT
LIFE	LIFE PATTERN & QUALITY	APOLLO	CREATIVITY, COMPASSION
HEART	EMOTIONAL NATURE	SATURN	INTROSPECTION, SERIOUS
APOLLO	CREATIVE ENERGY	JUPITER	SELF CONFIDENCE, LEADER
MERCURY	HEALTH, BUSINESS	LOWER MARS	OVERCOMING OBSTACLES, SELF CONTROL
SATURN	FATE, DESTINY	UPPER MARS	DETERMINATION, COURAGE
MARRIAGE	RELATIONSHIPS, FRIENDS	VENUS	PHYSICAL/SEXUAL ENERGY
		MOON	INTUITION, SENTIMENTAL

LINE TRAITS / ATTRIBUTES		MARKINGS / ATTRIBUTES	
FINE	SUBTLE PERCEPTION	BARS	INTERIM BARRIERS
DEEP	STRONG FEELINGS	BREAK INS	WEAKNESS
FEW, COARSE SKIN	PHYSICAL ENERGY	BRANCHES	EXTRA STRENGTH
FEW, DELICATE SKIN	INTUITIVE ENERGY	CIRCLES	AMPLIFY MIND/ BODY HEALTH
MANY	NERVOUS ENERGY	CROSSES	UPHEAVAL
DEEP MAIN LINES	DEEP FEELINGS	GRIDS	OBSTACLES
DEEP MAIN LINES/HIGH MOUNTS	PASSIONATE	ISLANDS	DELAYS, PROBLEMS
MAIN LINES IN BREAKS & CHAINS	PHYSICAL STRAIN	QUADRANGLES	ENHANCED PERSONAL TRAIT
PALE	LACK OF ENERGY	STARS	LUCK, SUCCESS
YELLOW LINES	NERVOUS, INHIBITED	SQUARES	STRENGTHEN WEAK AREA
RED LINES	STRONG FEELINGS	TASSELS	HINDRANCES
PINK WELL MARKED LINES	HEALTHY MIND & BODY	TRIANGLES	LUCK

PHRENOLOGY

AREA	PLANET	ASPECT	BUMP QUALITIES	AREA	PLANET	ASPECT	BUMP QUALITIES
1	MERCURY	INDIVIDUALITY	OBSERVATION DISCRIMINATION	22	JUPITER	HOPE	OPTIMISM
2	MERCURY	EVENTUALITY	MEMORY CURRENT EVENTS	23	JUPITER	IDEALITY	BEAUTY APPRECIATION REFINEMENT
3	MERCURY	COMPARISON	JUDGEMENT REASON	24	JUPITER	SUBLIMITY	LOVE OF THE BEST ROMANTIC. VIEWPOINT
4	MERCURY	CASUALITY	ORIGINALITY	25	SATURN	FIRMNESS	DETERMINATION EXERCISE OF WILL
5	MERCURY	MIRTH	HUMOR	26	SATURN	CONSCIENTIOUS	MORAL FIBER
6	MERCURY	LOCALITY	RECOLLECTION SENSE OF DIRECTION	27	SATURN	CAUTION	SELF PRESERVATION
7	MERCURY	TIME	RHYTHM REGULARITY	28	SATURN	SECRETIVE	RESERVE SELF RESTRAINT
8	MERCURY	TUNE	EAR FOR MUSIC	29	SUN	SELF ESTEEM	EGOTISM
9	MERCURY	CALCULATION	MATHEMATICAL ABILITY	30	SUN	APPROBATIVENESS	LOVE OF PRAISE DESIRE FOR APPROVAL
10	MERCURY	ORDER	ORGANIZATION	31	SUN	CONTINUITY	CONCENTRATION
11	MERCURY	COLOR	COLOR DISTINCTION	32	MARS	CONSTRUCTIVENESS	INVENTIVENESS CONSTRUCTIVE ACTION
12	MERCURY	WEIGHT	MOTION BALANCE	33	MARS	AQUISITIVENESS	ACCUMULATION
13	MERCURY	SIZE	OBJECT SIZE JUDGEMENT	34	MARS	ALIMENTIVENESS	FOOD METABOLISM SUSTENANCE
14	MERCURY	FORM	SHAPE JUDGEMENT	35	MARS	EXECUTION	ENDURANCE
15	MERCURY	LANGUAGE	ELOQUENCE	36	MARS	COMBATIVENESS	COURAGE AGGRESSION
16	JUPITER	HUMANITY	UNDERSTANDING	37	MARS	VITALITY	ZEST FOR LIFE ILLNESS RESISTANCE
17	JUPITER	BENEVOLENCE	SYMPATHY GENEROSITY	38	VENUS	FRIENDSHIP	FRIENDSHIP ABILITY SOCIAL AFFAIRS
18	JUPITER	VENERATION	REVERENCE RESPECT	39	VENUS	CONJUGALITY	MARITAL STATUS
19	JUPITER	AGREEABLENESS	POPULARITY	40	VENUS	AMATIVENESS	SENSUALITY SEX APPEAL
20	JUPITER	IMITATION	IMITATIVE ABILITY	41	MOON	INHABITIVENESS	HOME LIFE
21	JUPITER	SPIRITUALITY	FAITH RELIGIOUS FEELING	42	MOON	PARENTAL LOVE	LOVE OF CHILDREN

PHRENOLOGY

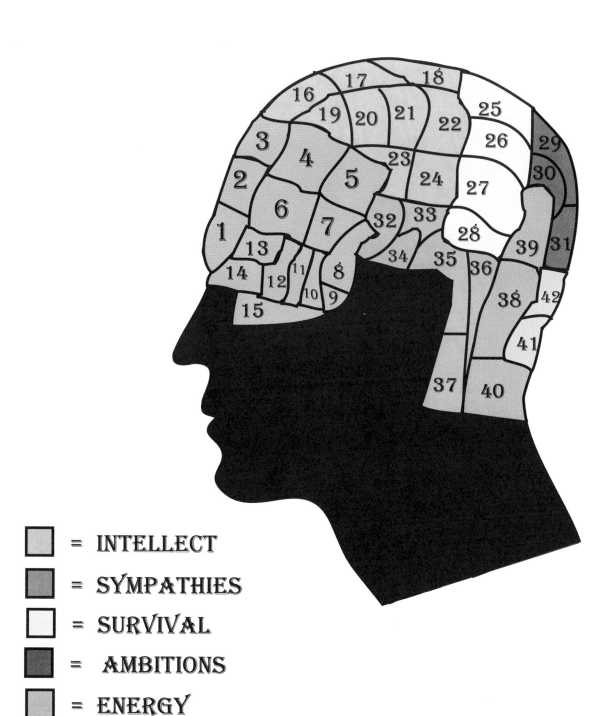

= INTELLECT

= SYMPATHIES

= SURVIVAL

= AMBITIONS

= ENERGY

= EMOTIONS

= SOCIAL INSTINCTS

PLANETS

PLANET	SIGN	MUSICAL NOTE	NUMBER	ASTRO HOUSE	RAY	ELEMENT/ POLARITY	SEPHIRAH	RULES
☉ SUN	LEO	D	1	5TH	2ND	FIRE POSITIVE	TIPHERETH (BEAUTY)	VITALITY SELF EXPRESSION LEADERSHIP CREATIVE POWERS
☽ MOON	CANCER	G SHARP, A FLAT	3, 9	4TH	4TH	WATER NEGATIVE	JESOD (FOUNDATION)	EMOTIONS WOMEN RELATIONSHIPS THE NIGHT WATER
☿ MERCURY	GEMINI	E	1, 4	3RD	4TH	AIR POSITIVE\ NEGATIVE	CHOD (GLORY)	COMMUNICATION INTELLIGENCE HUMOR, DEXTERITY SCIENCE, MEMORY
♀ VENUS	TAURUS LIBRA	F SHARP, G FLAT	5, 6, 7	2ND, 7TH	5TH	EARTH\AIR NEGATIVE	NETZACH (VICTORY)	LOVE, BEAUTY HARMONY, SEX SOCIABILITY PARTNERSHIPS MONEY
♂ MARS	ARIES	C	9	1ST	6TH	FIRE POSITIVE	GEBURAH (JUDGEMENT)	STRENGTH, STAMINA SHARP INSTRUMENTS ENERGY, FIRE PRODUCTIVITY MILITARY
♃ JUPITER	SAGITARRIUS	A SHARP, B FLAT	3	9TH, 12TH	2ND	FIRE POSITIVE	CHESED (MERCY)	ETHICS, TRUTH LUCK, PROSPERITY OPPORTUNITY LEGAL AFFAIRS
♄ SATURN	CAPRICORN	A	8	10TH, 11TH	3RD	EARTH POSITIVE	BINAH (UNDERSTANDING)	PATIENCE, REALISM RESPONSIBILITY STRUCTURE HISTORY, KARMA KNOWLEDGE
♅ URANUS	AQUARIUS	E	4	11TH	7TH	AIR POSITIVE	-	CHANGE, GENIUS INVENTION ELECTRICITY AVANT GARDE
♆ NEPTUNE	PISCES	G SHARP, A FLAT	7	12TH	6TH	WATER -	-	IMAGINATION MYSTICISM, RHTHYM UNCONSCIOUS SECRETS HIDDEN MEANINGS
♇ PLUTO	SCORPIO	C	-	8TH, 1ST	1ST	WATER -	-	DESTINY TRANSFORMATION ENERGY RECYCLING REINCARNATION

PLANETS

PLANET	DIAMETER (MILES)	DISTANCE FROM SUN MILLIONS OF MILES	POSITION NEAREST SUN	# SATELLITES	# DAYS ROTATION AROUND SUN	METAL	GEMSTONE
☉ SUN	864,000					TIGERS EYE TOPAZ ZIRCON	GOLD BRASS
☿ MERCURY	3,100	43.4M	1		88	FIRE OPAL CARNELIAN	WHITE ALLOY (NO TIN/SILVER)
♀ VENUS	7,543	67.7M	2		225	MALACHITE JADE CORAL AMBER	COPPER
⊕ EARTH	7,926	94.6M	3	1	365 DAYS 24 HOURS		
♂ MARS	4,200	155M	4	2	687 DAYS 24 HOURS 37 MINUTES	GARNET	IRON STEEL
♃ JUPITER	88,980	507M	5	16	4,332	LAPIS LAZULI AMETHYST	TIN
♄ SATURN	71,000	937M	6	16	10,760	ONYX JET	LEAD
♅ URANUS	32,000	1859.7M	7	5	30,684		
♆ NEPTUNE	30,600	2821.7M	8	2	60,188		
♇ PLUTO	1,680	4551.4M	9	1	90,467		

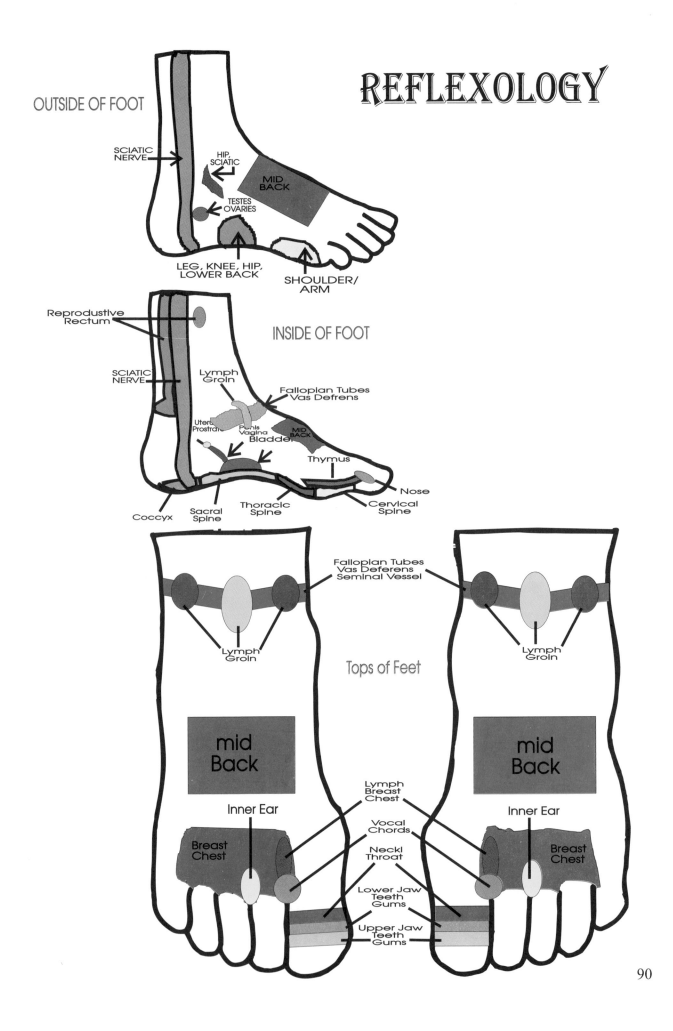

REFLEXOLOGY

OUTSIDE OF FOOT

SCIATIC NERVE

HIP, SCIATIC

MID BACK

TESTES OVARIES

LEG, KNEE, HIP, LOWER BACK

SHOULDER/ ARM

INSIDE OF FOOT

Reprodustive Rectum

SCIATIC NERVE

Lymph Groin

Fallopian Tubes Vas Defrens

Uteru Prostrat

Penis Vagina Bladder

MID BACK

Thymus

Nose

Cervical Spine

Thoracic Spine

Coccyx

Sacral Spine

Nose

Tops of Feet

Fallopian Tubes Vas Deferens Seminal Vessel

Lymph Groin

Lymph Groin

mid Back

mid Back

Lymph Breast Chest

Inner Ear

Inner Ear

Vocal Chords

Breast Chest

Neckl Throat

Breast Chest

Lower Jaw Teeth Gums

Upper Jaw Teeth Gums

90

REFLEXOLOGY

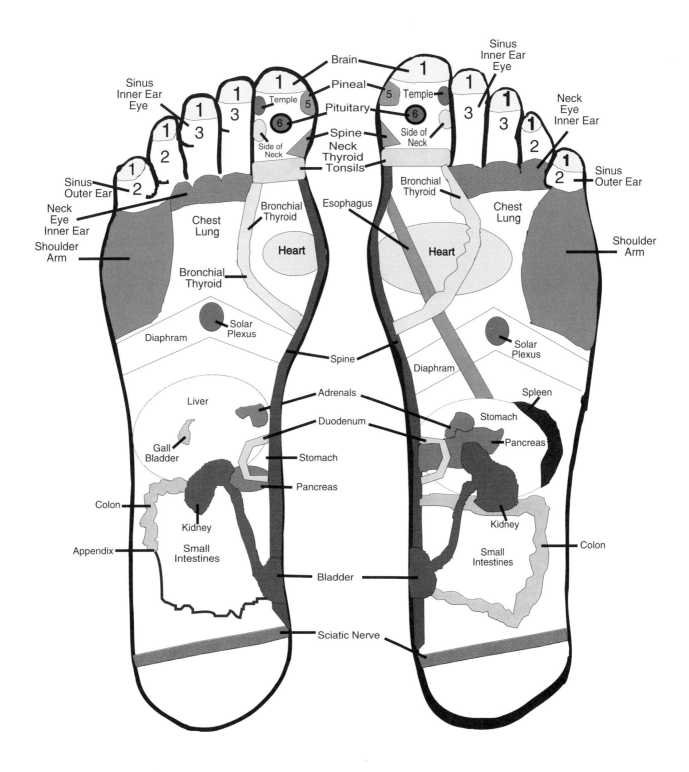

RUNES

SIGN	KEY WORD/ SYMBOL	GOD/ GODDESS	FIRE-WOOD	GEM	COLOR/ ELEMENT	OBJECT	METAL	MEANING
ᚠ FEOH	POSSESION / CATTLE				FIRE			DOMINION WEALTH POSSESION LUXURY
ᚢ UR	ACTION / AUROCHS				FIRE			FREEDOM COURAGE STRENGTH ACTION
ᚦ THORN	EVIL / DEVIL	LOKI	THORN	OPAL	GREY / WATER	SHOES	ARSENIC	ENVY CLEANSING NEMISIS PURGING
ᚩ OS	GOOD / GOD	ODIN	ASH	DIAMOND	WHITE / WATER	SPEAR	MERCURY	WISDOM TRUTH LOVE HEALTH
ᚱ RAD	JOURNEY / RIDING				AIR			TRAVEL EVOLUTION ESCAPE RELOCATION
ᚲ KEN	BEACON / TORCH				AIR			VISION CLARITY KNOWLEDGE REVELATION
ᚷ GYFU	GIFT / GIFT				EARTH			GIFT BEQUEST LEGACY OFFERING
ᚹ WYN	HAPPINESS / GLORY				EARTH			JOY ECSTASY LEGACY BLISS
ᚺ HAEGL	HARDSHIP / HAIL				FIRE			TEMPERING REBUILDING TESTING TRIAL
ᚾ NYD	NECESSITY / NEED				FIRE			NECESSITY WANT NEED TORMENT
ᛁ IS	ENTRAPMENT / ICE	HEL	WILLOW	JET	BLACK / WATER	VEIL	LEAD	GLAMOUR ALLURE INFATUATION INVITATION
ᛃ GER	CHANGE / HARVEST				WATER			CHANGE ALTERATION LUCK FRUITION

RUNES

SIGN	KEY/SYMBOL	GOD/GODDESS	FIRE-WOOD	GEM	COLOR/ELEMENT	OBJECT	METAL	MEANING
EOH	DUTY / YEW	HEIMDALL	YEW	SAPPHIRE	BLUE / AIR	HORN	STEEL	TRUTH RELIABLE STRENGTH TENACITY
PEROD	PLEASURE / APPLE	FRIJA	APPLE	EMERALD	GREEN / AIR	NECKLACE	COPPER	ABUNDANCE SENSUALITY OPULENCE LUXURY
EOLH	PROTECTION / DEFENSE				EARTH			PROTECTION SHIELD DEFENSE GUARDIAN
SIGEL	RETRIBUTION / SUN	THOR	OAK	JASPER	ORANGE / EARTH	HAMMER	TIN	POWER ENERGY ACT OF WILL FORCE
TYR	JUDGEMENT / TIW	TIW	FIR	RUBY	RED / FIRE	SWORD	IRON	VICTORY VALOR HONOR INTEGRITY
BEORC	FERTILITY / BIRCH	FREYJA	BIRCH	AMETHYST	PURPLE / FIRE	CLOAK	SILVER	LOVE GROWTH HEALING FERTILITY
EH	TRANSPORTATION / HORSE				WATER			GRACE SPEED MOVEMENT TRANSPORTATION
MAN	INTELLEGENCE / MAN				WATER			INVENTION SKILL ABILITY INTELLIGENCE
LAGU	UNCONSCIOUS / WATER				AIR			MYSTERY HISTORY DREAMS FANTASIES
ING	GROWTH / FERTILITY				AIR			STABILITY CARING FAMILY GOOD SENSE
DAEG	COMPLETION / DAY	BALDER	MISTLETOE	TOPAZ	YELLOW / EARTH	BOW	GOLD	REBIRTH PERIOD CYCLE PHASE
ETHEL	HOME / HOMELAND	FREY	PINE	AGATE	RED BROWN / EARTH	CHARIOT	BRONZE	PATRIOTISM KARMA HOME PROPERTY

THE SEVEN RAYS

TWO RAYS DOMINATE EACH LIFE. ONE RAY FOR THE SOUL, AND THE OTHER FOR THE PERSONALITY.

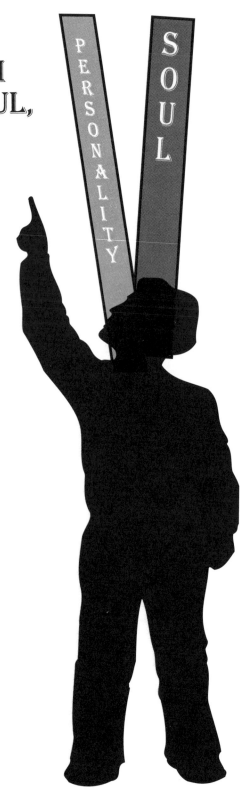

THE SEVEN RAYS

RAY	ASTROLOGY	SYMBOL	COLOR	PHRASE	POLARITY
1	TAURUS PISCES	THE FATHER	RED	CREATIVITY WILL	POSITIVE
2	LEO SAGITTARIUS AQUARIUS	THE SON	LIGHT BLUE	LOVE WISDOM TRUTH	NEGATIVE
3	CAPRICORN SAGITTARIUS	THE HOLY SPIRIT	YELLOW	INTELLIGENCE HARMONY	POSITIVE
4	VIRGO, CANCER GEMINI, ARIES	THE HAND OF GOD	GREEN	BEAUTY PASSION	NEGATIVE
5	GEMINI LIBRA TAURUS	THE MIND OF GOD	ORANGE	KNOWLEDGE	POSITIVE
6	CANCER ARIES SCORPIO	JESUS THE MAN	INDIGO	DEVOTION IDEALISM	NEGATIVE
7	AQUARIUS LIBRA	UNVEILED MAGICIAN	VIOLET	MAGIC CEREMONY	POSITIVE

SIOUX
FOUR DIRECTIONS

N

W

E

S

SIOUX
FOUR DIRECTIONS

DIRECTION	LIFE STAGE	HOUSE	COLOR	ANIMAL	RELATION
EAST	OLD AGE DEATH AFTER LIFE	MORNING STAR	YELLOW	DOVE GOLDEN EAGLE	WISDOM UNDERSTANDING
SOUTH	BIRTH	ANIMAL SPIRITS	WHITE	DEER WHITE CRANE	LIFE DESTINY
WEST	YOUTH	THUNDER	BLACK	BUFFALO BLACK EAGLE	PURIFYING WATER
NORTH	MIDDLE AGE	CALF PIPE WOMAN	RED	BALD EAGLE	HEALTH

THE TAROT

CARD/NUMBER	QUALITIES	LIFE CYCLE	MUSIC NOTE	CHAKRA	ASTOLOGY/PLANETS	MEANING	ARCHETYPE
THE FOOL 0	ORIGIN/END CONTINGENCY IMPULSE/CHAOS	EMBRYO HUMAN	E	3RD EYE TO CROWN	URANUS	FACING THE UNKNOWN CHANGE IN DIRECTION THE UNEXPECTED	DIONYSUS CAIN ORESTES
THE JUGGLER 1	WILL CREATIVITY INTUITION	CHILDHOOD HUMAN	E	3RD EYE TO CROWN	MERCURY	NEW VITALITY NEW OPPORTUNITIES INTUITIVE POWER	HERMES ADAM
HIGH PRIESTESS 2	BODY HEALING WISDOM MYSTERY	CHILDHOOD HUMAN	G SHARP A FLAT	HEART TO CROWN	MOON	MOTHER NATURE DISCOVERY INNER SELF HIGHLY INTUITIVE	MOIRA ISIS DIANA
EMPRESS 3	EARTHINESS NATURE FECUNDITY	CHILDHOOD HUMAN	F SHARP G FLAT	3RD EYE	VENUS	MARRIAGE PARTNERSHIP CREATIVE PERIOD	APHRODITE DEMETER EARTH MOTHER
EMPEROR 4	MASCULINE MIND/WILL DIRECTION CONSCIOUS ENERGY	CHILDHOOD HUMAN	C	NAVEL TO SOLAR	ARIES	EVALUATE REFORM AUTHORITY STRUCTURE	ZEUS THOR JEHOVAH
HIGH PRIEST 5	SOUL HEALING SELF DISCOVERY UNDERSTANDING	CHILDHOOD HUMAN	C SHARP D FLAT	NAVEL TO SOLAR	TAURUS	RELIGION INTELLIGENCE METAPHYSICS	HE (THE BREATH)
THE LOVERS 6	SOCIETY MORALITY CONFER RIGHTS	CHILDHOOD HUMAN	D	THROAT TO 3RD EYE	GEMINI	LOVE CHOICE CAREER CHOICE	DIOSCURI PARIS
THE CHARIOT 7	POWER INTELLECT SELF CONFIDENCE	CHILDHOOD HUMAN	D SHARP E FLAT	THROAT TO 3RD EYE	CANCER	BALANCE INTELLIGENCE CONTROL OF PASSION	ARES
JUSTICE 8	REASON BALANCE OF WILL	CHILDHOOD HUMAN	F SHARP G FLAT	HEART TO THROAT	LIBRA	MAKE DECISION GIVE & TAKE BALANCE PERCEPTION	ATHENA PALLAS
THE HERMIT 9	ISOLATION ROOTLESSNESS STOIC WISDOM	CHILDHOOD HUMAN	F	HEAD TO THROAT	VIRGO	BUILD FOUNDATION PATIENCE FIND HIGHER NEED	KRONOS BUDDHA MARCUS AURELIUS
WHEEL OF FORTUNE 10	IDEAL FORM CHANCE FATE	CHILDHOOD HUMAN	A SHARP B FLAT	SOLAR	JUPITER	CHANGE OF FATE NEW GROWTH	THE FURIES
STRENGTH 11	NATURE TAMER POWER MIRACLE	CHILDHOOD HUMAN	E	SOLAR	LEO	COURAGE STRENGTH DISCIPLINE	HERCULES RICHARD THE LION HEARTED

THE TAROT

CARD/ NUMBER	QUALITIES	LIFE CYCLE	MUSIC NOTE	CHAKRA	ASTOLOGY/ PLANETS	MEANING	ARCHETYPE
THE HANGED MAN 12	SACRIFICE PATIENT VIRTUE HARDEN WILL	CHILDHOOD HUMAN	G SHARP A FLAT	SOLAR TO THROAT	NEPTUNE	ATTITUDE FANTASY PRUDENCE	PROMETHEUS
DEATH 13	TRANSFORMATION	ADOLESCENT COSMIC	G	SOLAR TO HEART	SCORPIO	PASSAGE TO CYCLE	PLUTO JUDAS
TEMPERANCE 14	PERSONIFIED VIRTUES SUPERNATURAL	ADOLESCENT COSMIC	G SHARP A FLAT	NAVEL TO HEART	SAGITTARIUS	ACCESS BALANCE ADAPTING RELATIONSHIP	IRIS
THE DEVIL 15	LIBIDO REBEL WILL	ADOLESCENT COSMIC	A	SOLAR TO HEART	CAPRICORN	UNNECESSARY TIES TO MATERIAL WORLD COFRONTING OTHER SIDE	PAN CEREBUS
THE TOWER 16	ENDING BLIND FAITH INTROSPECTIVE THOUGHT	ADOLESCENT COSMIC	C	SOLAR TO HEART	MARS	STORM BEFORE CALM DISRUPTION THROUGH INTELLECT	KING MINOS
THE STAR 17	MEDIATION ENLIGHTENMENT	ADOLESCENT COSMIC	A SHARP B FLAT	HEART TO 3RD EYE	AQUARIUS	HOPE INSPIRATION HEALTH	PANDORA
THE MOON 18	BOUND SPIRIT COMPROMISE ILLUSION OF MATTER	ADOLESCENT COSMIC	B	ROOT TO SOLAR	PISCES	UNCERTAINITY MANY MEANINGS INSTINCT	HECATE
THE SUN 19	JOY, HOPE FREEDOM REGAINED INNOCENCE	ADOLESCENT COSMIC	D	NAVEL TO SOLAR	THE SUN	WORLDLY DEEDS GOOD RELATIONSHIP CLARITY, TRUST	ATEN APOLLO
THE LAST JUDGEMENT 20	FUTURE CONSCIOUSNESS	ADOLESCENT COSMIC	C	ROOT TO SOLAR	PLUTO	SPIRITUAL AWAKENING RENEWAL CONSCIOUS SHIFT	HESTIA HERMES
THE WORLD 21	ETERNITY CONCRETE ACTUALITY	ADOLESCENT COSMIC	A	ROOT TO NAVEL	SATURN	FULLFILLMENT HARMONY	KALI SOPHIA

TEA LEAF READING

SYMBOL	TYPE	MEANING	SYMBOL	TYPE	MEANING
Anchor	+	Unsettled Condition	Money	Neutral	Money
Angel	+	Protection, Awareness	Moon	Neutral	Change
Ape	+	Mimic, Copy	Mountain	+	Challenge
Baby	Neutral	New Venture or Start	Mouse	-	Pest
Balloon	+	Fun, Take Chance	Music Note	+	Harmony
Banana	+	Foreign Interaction	Necktie	-	Conformity
Bat	Neutral	Treachery, Danger	Nest	Neutral	Emotional Security
Bell	-	Announcement	Pig	-	Greed
Bird	Neutral	Good Message	Pipe	+	Reconciliation
Blobs	Neutral	Ordinary Next Year	Power Lines	+	Great Resources
Bottle	Neutral	Temptation	Rabbit	+	Carefree
Cane	-	Temporary Illness	Rainbow	+	Easy Going
Clouds	Neutral	Temporary Problem	Rake	-	Search
Diamond	+	Jewelry, Gift	Ring	+	Marriage
Dish	Neutral	Invitation	Rope	Neutral	Capture
Door	+	Opportunity	SeaHorse	+	Family
Ear	+	Good News	Sheep	+	Passive
Egg	+	Success	Shoe	+	Effort
Eye	+	Psychic Ability	Skeleton	-	A Secret
Fish	+	Increased Wealth	Spider	+	Good Luck
Flag	Neutral	Maintain Integrity	Spoon	+	Training
Flowers	+	Compliments	Stairs	+	Success
Foot	+	New Experience	Star	+	Success
Fork	+	Assistance	Sun	+	Happiness
Glass	Neutral	Dissatisfaction	Table	+	Favor
Gun	Neutral	Anger	Tear Drop	-	Sorrow
Hand	+	Assistance	Telephone	+	Business Meeting
Hat	+	New Role	Telescope	Neutral	Long Distance Call
Heart	+	Love	Torch	Neutral	Sacrifice
Hills	+	Truth	Tree	+	Family
Horseshoe	+	Good Luck	Truck	+	Hardwork
Jug	+	Party	Umbrella	+	Protection
Kettle	Neutral	Guests	Vase	+	Secret Admirer
Key	+	Success	Wall	-	Misunderstanding
Knife	-	Fear	Whale	-	Worry Over Nothing
Ladder	+	Success	Wine Glass	+	Party
Lamb	+	Kindness	Worm	+	Humility
Lamp	+	Guidance	Wreath	-	Sorrow
Leaf	Neutral	Health	Wishbone	+	Wish Granted

TEA LEAF READING

Tea Cup Preparation

1) 1/2 teaspoon loose tea in cup, pour hot water, drink..
2) Leave small bit of water at bottom and swirl cup.
3) Rotate cup at an angle to slosh out water.
4) Turn cup over on paper towel in front of person.
5) Person rotates cup clockwise 3 times. (cup is still turned over)
6) Turn cup right side up. Do reading.

Position of Tea Leaves

Read Clockwise.
Look for Symbols.
2 Symbols 1/4" apart influence each other.

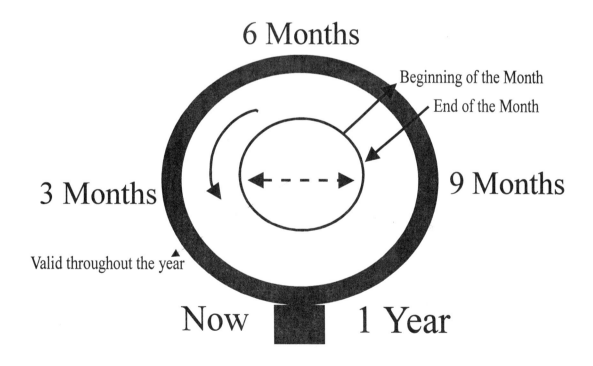

VITAMINS, MINERALS & SUPPLEMENTS

NAME	ACTIVITY	USES
A BETA CAROTENE	New Cell Growth. Fights Infection. Antioxidant.	Essential to Skin, Bones and Blood.
B1 THIAMINE	Metabolizes Sugar and Salt. Nervous System.	Large Amount - Diabetes Small Amount-Hypoglocemia
B2 RIBOFLAVIN	Good Muscle Tone. Metabolism of Fats, Protein and Carbohydrates.	Important to Vision, Skin, Hair and Nails.
B3 NIACIN	Nervous & Digestive Systems, Skin.	Healthy Skin.
B5 PANOTOTHENIC ACID	Energy, Hormone & Antibody Production.	Strengthens Adrenal Activity.
B6 PYRODOXINE	Energy Production. Utilizes Fats and Protein.	Large Amount - Diabetes
B12 CYANOCOBALAMIN	Builds Blood. Brain/Nervous System	Large Amount-Hypoglocemia
BIOTIN B COMP.	Produces Energy. Metabolizes Fats.	Forms RNA,DNA and Synthesizes Amino Acids.
C ASCORBIC ACID	Antioxidant, Collagen and Red Blood Cell Production. Aids Clotting.	Aids Immune System, Blood Cells, Cholesterol. Antibacterial.
CALCIUM	Strong Bones & Teeth. Essential for Heart Rhythm.	Aids Clotting, Thyroid, Adrenals. Calms Nerves.
CHOLINE B COMP.	Neurotransmitter. Aids Kidneys and Bladder.	Aids Nerve Fibers, Slows Fast Pulse Rate. Aids Digestion.
CHROMIUM	Glucose Metabolism. Synthesis Fatty Acids and Cholesterol.	Large Amount-Diabetes Small Amount-Hypoglocemia
CO-Q10 UBIQUINONE	Immune System, Energy, Cell Oxygen Level. Helps Over Weight.	Tissue Healing, Aids Angina, Hypertension, Vascular Disease.
COPPER	Aids Hemoglobin, Red Blood Cells, and Bone Formation.	Thyroid, Hormone, Adrenal Function. Calcium Utilization.
D CALCIFEROL	Aids Weak Muscles, Utilizes Calcium & Phosphorous.	Large Amount-Diabetes Small Amount-Hypoglocemia
DMG N, N-DIMETHYLGLYCINE	Reduces Seizures, Glucose Metabolism, Helps Liver Increase B & T Lymphocytes	AntiViral. Detoxifier. Increases Interferon. Antioxidant.
E MIXED TOCOPHEROLS	Antioxidant. Oxygen to Muscles. Protects Hormone Membranes.	Prolongs Red Blood Cell Life. Aids Proper Clotting.
EVENING PRIMROSE OIL	Essential Fatty Acid. Aids in Hormone Production.	Proper Organ Function.
FOLIC ACID B COMP.	Synthesizes Nucleo Proteins (RNA,DNA)	Needed for Red Blood Cells

VITAMINS, MINERALS & SUPPLEMENTS

NAME	ACTIVITY	USES
GARLIC	Helps Immune System. AntibBacterial.	Reduces Blood Pressure.
GERMANIUM GE 132	Aids Cell Function. Efficient Oxygen Antioxidant.	Anti-Arthritic. Anti-Tumor. AntiViral.
l-CYSTEINE AMINO ACID	Aids Immune System. Antibacterial. AntiViral.	Wound Healing. Aids Chelation of Heavy Body Metals.
l-GLUTAMINE GLUTAMIC ACID	High Level Brain Activity Source.	Lessen Mental Fatigue.
l-LYSINE AMINO ACID	AntiViral. Builds Antibodies.	Builds New Tissue. Aids Hormones.
l-PHENYLALANINE AMINO ACID	Decrease Pain. Antidepressant. Stimulates Pituitary.	Aids Endorphin Production.
INOSITOL B COMP.	Fat Metabolism. Hair Growth.	Brain Cell Nutrition.
IRON FERROUS SULPHATE	Hemoglobin Production.	Large Amount - Diabetes Small Amount - Hypoglocemia
LECITHIN	Aids Digestion and Cholesterol.	Prevents Infection, Gall Stones and Fatty Liver.
MAGNESIUM	Nerve Functions.	Bone Maintenance
MANGANESE	Protein & Fat Utilization. Maintains Nervous System.	Aids Sex Hormone Production.
MAX EPA	Cell Membrane Fomation. Lowers Cholesterol.	Used by Brain Nerve Fibers.
P BIOFLAVONIDS, RUTIN, HESPERIDIN	Part of C Complex.	Enhances Vitamin C.
PABA B COMP.	Forms Red Blood Cells. Utilization of Fats and Carbohydrates.	Hair Pigmentation.
PHOSPHORUS	Cell Maintenance.	Aids Nerve Conduction.
POTASSIUM	Heart Rhythm. Nerve Conduction.	Balance of Minerals in the Blood.
SELENIUM	Antioxidant	Aids Body Growth & Metabolism.
SOD COMPLEX SUPEROXIDE DISMUTASE, CATALASE, GLUTATHIONE PEROXIDASE	Neutralizes Free Radicals. Aids in Radiation Protection.	Lessens Emotional, Physical, Chemical & Nutritional Stress.
ZINC	Healing & Normal Growth Necessity. Aids New Cell Development.	Normal Function of Prostrate Gland.

WESTERN ELEMENTS

ELEMENT	DIRECTION	PLANETS	MOTIVATION	TREE	COLOR	NUMBERS	QUALITIES
FIRE	SOUTH	MARS JUPITER SUN	INSPIRATION	ALMOND	RED ORANGE GOLD	1, 3, 4, 9	ZEAL COURAGE CREATIVITY
EARTH	NORTH	VENUS SATURN	PHYSICAL	OAK	WHITE BROWN GREEN BLACK	5, 6, 8	NATURE DEPENDABLE CAUTIOUS
AIR	EAST	MERCURY VENUS URANUS	MENTAL	ASPEN	YELLOW RED WHITE	4, 5, 6	CURIOUS LOGICAL PERCEPTIVE
WATER	WEST	MOON PLUTO NEPTUNE	EMOTIONAL	WILLOW	GREEN GREY BLUE	2, 3, 7, 9	PSYCHIC SENSITIVE RECEPTIVE

WESTERN ELEMENTS

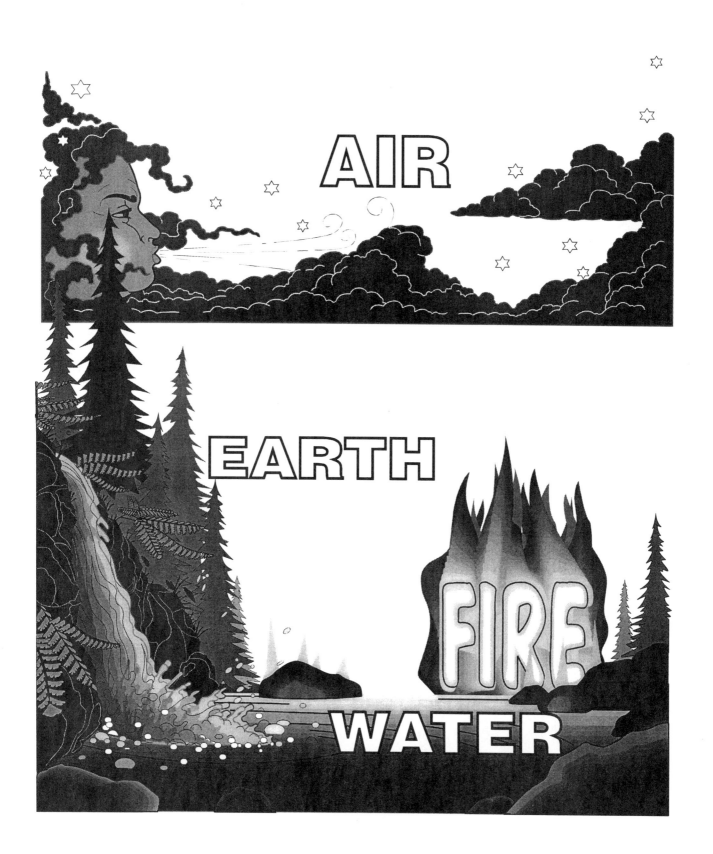

Reading List

Atwood, Mary Dean. *Spirit Healing*. New York: Sterling Publishing Co.

Bauer, Cathryn. *Acupressure for Everybody*. New York: Henry Holt & Co.

Bergman, Deborah. *Inner Voyager*. New York: Roundtable Press

Brown, Wensell. *How to Tell Fortunes with Cards*. New York: Bell Publishing

Davidson, Gustav. *A Dictionary of Angels*. New York: The Free Press

Domin, Linda. *Palmascope*. St. Paul, MN: Llewyellen Publications

Gimbutas, Marija. *Language of the Goddess*. New York: Harper & Row

Goodman, Linda. *Linda Goodman's Sun Signs*. New York: Bantam Books

Hawks, Wendy. *Oriental Horoscope*. Boca Raton, FL: Globe Communications Co.

Jackson, Joseph and Baument, John. *Pictorial Guide to Planets*. New York: Harper & Row

Kuthumi and Kuj, Djawal. *The Human Aura*. Malibu, CA: Summit University Press

Leek, Sybil. *Phrenology*. New York: Macmillan Company

Lewi, Grant. *Heaven Knows What*. St Paul, MN: Llewellyn Publications

Melody. *Love is in the Earth, A Kaleidscope of Crystals*. Wheatridge, CO: Earth-Love Press

Mysteries of the Unknown - Richmond, VA: Time/Life Books

Norman, Laura with Cowan, Thomas. *Feet First*. New York: Fireside

Ronner, John. *Know Your Angels*. Marlsboro, TN: Mamre Press

Santillo, Humbert. *Natural Healing with Herbs*. Prescott Valley, AZ: Hohm Press

Sawtell, Vanda. *The Medicine of the Stars*. London, England: Essential Nutrients, Ltd.

Tierra, Michael. *Way of Herbs*. New York: Pocket Books

Tyson, Daniel. *Rune Magic*. St. Paul, MN: Llewyellen Publications

Ussher, Arland. *The Twenty-Two Keys of the Tarot*. Dublin, Ireland: Dolman Press

Walker, Dr. Morton. *The Power of Color*. Garden City Park, NY: Avery Publishing Group

Wing, R.L. *The Illustrated I Ching*. New York: Doubleday

INDEX

Personal Notes

Personal Notes

Creative Health & Spirit

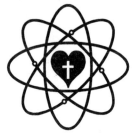

We hope you enjoyed this book and that it gives you many hours of fun and self-discovery. We appreciate your purchase of a Creative Health & Spirit book or product. Your investment allows Creative Health & Spirit to give free seminars on Visualization Healing to senior citizens and allows us to supply Alternative Medicine and Awareness information to the general public.

Creative Health & Spirit, an Alternative Medicine & Awareness company, specializes in providing products, services and information. We hope our products and services give you the tools you need to help you grow, maintain hope and feel good. Your satisfaction is the ultimate objective, for only by fulfilling your needs will we feel successful.

If you would like to order a catalog describing the numerous Alternative Medicine and Awareness gift items, audiovisualization self-healing tapes and services available to you from Creative Health & Spirit
or
If you have a comment, question or recommendation that you would like to share with Linda Mackenzie, please write or call us at:

Creative Health & Spirit
P.O. Box 385
Manhattan Beach, CA 90267
(800) 555-5453

"Lighting the Way with Energy, God & Love."